PRESS HERE!!

REIKI

~ FOR BEGINNERS ~

PRESS HERE!

REIKI

~ FOR BEGINNERS ~

YOUR GUIDE TO SUBTLE ENERGY THERAPY

VICTOR ARCHULETA

FAIR WINDS

Inspiring | Educating | Creating | Entertaining

Brimming with creative inspiration, how-to projects, and useful information to enrich your everyday life, Quarto Knows is a favorite destination for those pursuing their interests and passions. Visit our site and dig deeper with our books into your area of interest: Quarto Creates, Quarto Cooks, Quarto Homes, Quarto Lives, Quarto Drives, Quarto Explores, Quarto Gifts, or Quarto Kids.

First Published in 2017 by Fair Winds Press, an imprint of The Quarto Group. 100 Cummings Center, Suite 265-D, Beverly, MA 01915, USA T (978) 282-9590 F (978) 283-2742

Fair Winds Press titles are also available at discount for retail, wholesale, promotional, and bulk purchase. For details, contact the Special Sales Manager by email at specialsales@quarto.com or by mail at The Quarto Group, Attn: Special Sales Manager, 401 Second Avenue North, Suite 310, Minneapolis, MN 55401, USA.

21 20 19 18 17 1 2 3 4 5

ISBN: 978-1-59233-791-0

Digital edition published in 2017

QUAR.REIK

Conceived, designed, and produced by Quarto Publishing plc. 6 Blundell Street, London N7 9BH

Editor: Kate Burkett
Senior art editor: Emma Clayton
Designer and Illustrator: Emily Portnoi
Art director: Caroline Guest
Creative director: Moira Clinch
Publisher: Samantha Warrington

Printed in China

The information in this book is for educational purposes only. It is not intended to replace the advice of a physician or medical practitioner. Please see your health-care provider before beginning any new health program.

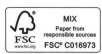

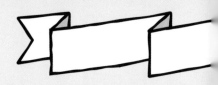

CONTENTS

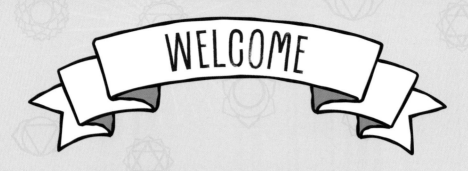

WELCOME

REIKI—LIKE SUBTLE ENERGY THERAPY PROVIDES CALM, SOOTHING COMFORT THAT MAY HELP TO RELIEVE PAIN, STRESS, AND ANXIETY AND OFFER REASSURANCE AND SUPPORT FOR PHYSICAL, MENTAL, AND ENERGETIC DISEASE CAUSED BY MANY TYPES OF TRAUMATIC EXPERIENCES.

THE BUSY AND SOMETIMES FRENETIC PACE OF 21ST—CENTURY LIVING CAN MAKE IT CHALLENGING TO MAINTAIN BALANCE AND CLARITY IN OUR EVERYDAY LIVES. WE TRY TO DO IT ALL, BUT IT CAN OFTEN BE AN UPHILL BATTLE. SURE, WE CAN BE SUPER ORGANIZED AND DISCIPLINED TO ACCOMPLISH EVERYTHING WE WANT TO ACHIEVE, AND OFTEN SUCCEED IN DOING SO, BUT SOMETIMES WE FALL SHORT.

BY MAKING A COMMITMENT TO OUR WELLNESS AND
THE WELLNESS OF OTHERS, WE CAN ACTUALLY ACHIEVE
MORE OF OUR GOALS WITH GRACE AND EASE IN A
BALANCED AND FOCUSED WAY. THE READER CAN UTILIZE
THE EASY—TO—USE TOOLS PRESENTED IN THIS BOOK TO
HELP THEMSELVES AND THEIR LOVED ONES AS PART OF
AN OVERALL WELLNESS PLAN.

VICTOR ARCHULETA

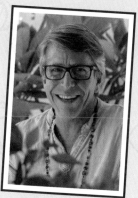

DISCLAIMER

The information presented in this book is not intended as a substitute
for training by a reiki master and the methodologies and protocols
presented should only be utilized as a gift to the readers themselves and
to their loved ones. If you are inspired by what you learn here, you are
encouraged to seek out a local reiki master to lead you through the
attunement process so that you can fully utilize this powerful tool.

THE BENEFITS OF REIKI

Subtle Energy Therapy is effective, safe, gentle, non-invasive, and easy to use. It might prove effective in:

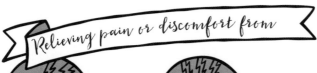

Relieving pain or discomfort from

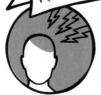

HEADACHES

MIGRAINES

NECK PAIN

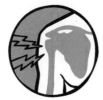

SHOULDER PAIN

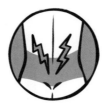

LOWER BACK PAIN

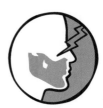

JAW PAIN

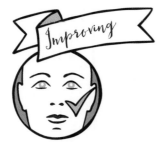

Improving

CLARITY AND FOCUS

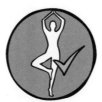

FLEXIBILITY AND RANGE OF MOTION

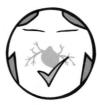

YOUR OVERALL WELL-BEING

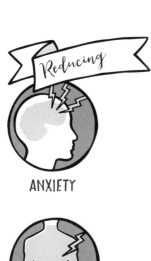

ANXIETY

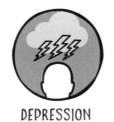

DEPRESSION

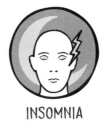

INSOMNIA

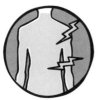
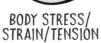

BODY STRESS/
STRAIN/TENSION

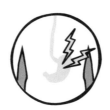

DIGESTIVE IRREGULARITY

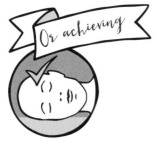

DEEP RELAXATION

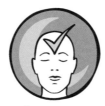

DEEP/RESTFUL SLEEP

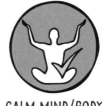

CALM MIND/BODY

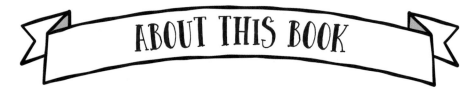

ABOUT THIS BOOK

This contemporary take on a traditional practice makes Reiki accessible to a new generation of readers. Beautiful illustrations, the expertise of teacher and practitioner Victor Archuleta, and simple step-by-step protocols allow readers to learn this fun and powerful wellness tool.

CHAPTER 1

Your Reiki Session

Reiki energy work depends on focused intention and willingness —the intention of the "sender" to invoke the flow of energy and the willingness of the "receiver" to accept the energy flow. This chapter teaches you how to access this energy by centering yourself and meditating on Reiki principles and affirmations as well as a step-by-step guide to plan, prepare, and perform your session.

PRELIMINARY STEPS
FOUR PREPARATORY
STEPS BEFORE STARTING
YOUR SESSION ARE
EXPLAINED IN DETAIL

ILLUSTRATIONS
VISUALS ILLUSTRATE
HOW TO ACCESS THE
ENERGY REQUIRED FOR
YOUR SESSION

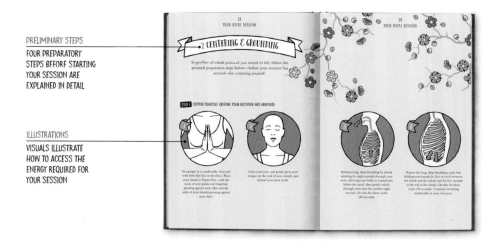

CHAPTER 2

Traditional Hand Positions

In this hands-on chapter, you will learn the principles and methods of using the standard Reiki hand positions for overall well-being. This chapter will teach you how to use these hand positions to influence subtle energy flow in some of the particular energy centers and meridians also used in Chinese acupuncture. You will learn 15 hand positions for a self-help protocol and 15 for family-help protocol.

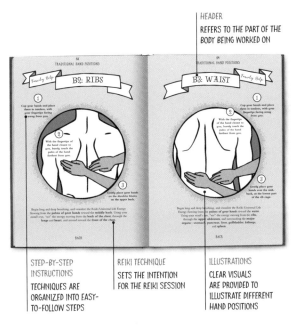

HEADER
REFERS TO THE PART OF THE BODY BEING WORKED ON

STEP-BY-STEP INSTRUCTIONS
TECHNIQUES ARE ORGANIZED INTO EASY-TO-FOLLOW STEPS

REIKI TECHNIQUE
SETS THE INTENTION FOR THE REIKI SESSION

ILLUSTRATIONS
CLEAR VISUALS ARE PROVIDED TO ILLUSTRATE DIFFERENT HAND POSITIONS

CHAPTER 3

Ailment Categories for Specific Symptoms

Often there is a need to address a specific symptom or ailment. This chapter will provide three possible options to approach your Reiki session for a specific symptom or ailment. This chapter will also explain how you can first determine which ailment category type—by physical location, by body system, or by chakra—you think is most appropriate. Step-by-step instructions are then provided for each category that can be used to learn the specific protocol needed to achieve your goal.

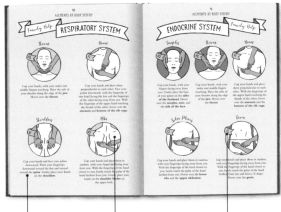

INSTRUCTIONS
DETAILED INSTRUCTIONS EXPLAIN WHERE TO PLACE HANDS TO SEEK RELIEF FROM PAIN

ILLUSTRATIONS
A SEQUENCE OF VISUALS IS GIVEN TO PROVIDE RELIEF FOR A SPECIFIC AILMENT

LABELS
CROSS REFER BACK TO HAND POSITIONS IN CHAPTER 2

KEY					
H HEAD	H1 EYES	F1 HEART	B1 SHOULDERS	L1 KNEE
F FRONT	H2 TEMPLES	F2 SOLAR	B2 RIBS	L2 ANKLE
B BACK	H3 SKULL	PLEXUS	B3 WAIST	L3 SOLE
L LEGS/FEET	H4 THROAT	F3 NAVEL	B4 COCCYX	
		F4 GROIN		

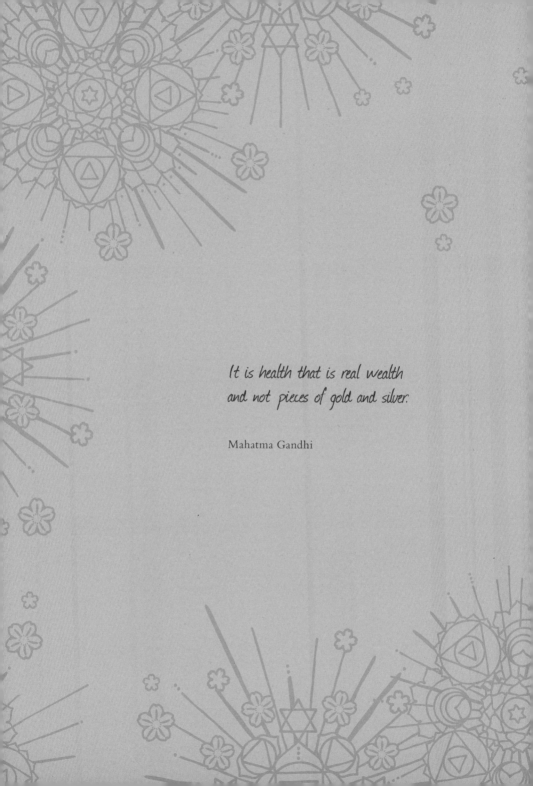

It is health that is real wealth
and not pieces of gold and silver.

Mahatma Gandhi

1

YOUR REIKI SESSION

WHAT IS REIKI & HOW IT WORKS

Reiki is Japanese for "Universal Life Energy," and it is the word used to describe a system of natural healing. Reiki is a noninvasive approach to wellness that was developed to improve overall well-being. Through the intention of the "sender" and the willingness of the "receiver"—and the use of specific hand positions—subtle energy transfer can be used to facilitate flow in the body. The energy flows from the palms of the hands of the sender to influence the energy flow of the receiver.

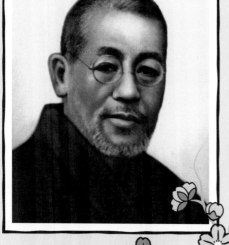

History

Traditional Reiki was originally developed and practiced in the early 1900s by Mikao Usui in Japan. In Reiki practice, energy is transferred to the recipient by laying the hands on or near the body to promote healing and well-being and to alleviate stress. Today Reiki is extremely popular in the West.

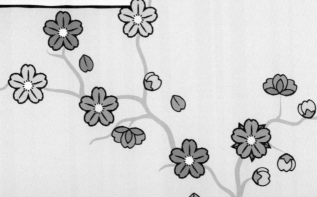

REIKI PRINCIPLES

The power inherent in subtle energy work is not dependent on a belief or understanding; it's more of a trusting and allowing of the process to unfold. Practicing the fundamental principles of Reiki provides a foundation from which the work can progress.

Five principles that guide this work are included in the Reiki Prayer:

Just for today...

I LET GO OF ANGER

I LET GO OF WORRY

I AM GRATEFUL

I WORK ON MYSELF

I AM KIND TO ALL LIVING THINGS

The space that you create for yourself as a sender, and your friend or family member as the receiver, is not only a physical space, it is also an energetic and perhaps even spiritual space. It is the container in which the work can occur.

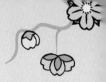

PLANNING YOUR SESSION

Before starting to practice, determine whether you'd like to
address an issue with yourself or someone else, and determine
if you are addressing something specific or whether you would
like to do a session for overall well-being.

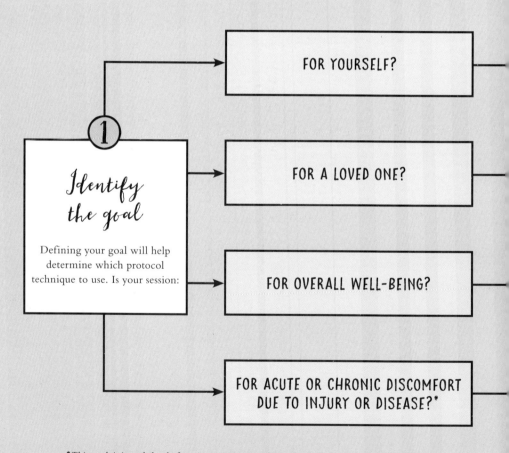

①

*Identify
the goal*

Defining your goal will help
determine which protocol
technique to use. Is your session:

FOR YOURSELF?

FOR A LOVED ONE?

FOR OVERALL WELL-BEING?

**FOR ACUTE OR CHRONIC DISCOMFORT
DUE TO INJURY OR DISEASE?***

*This work is intended only for minor injuries, i.e., skin or bones that are not broken. It is very
important to seek the aid of a medical professional immediately if you are not sure of the severity
of the injury. Do not rely on Subtle Energy Therapy alone to address a serious injury.

③

Find your protocol

Once you know which approach you would like to take and the specific area you'd like to address, you can then go directly to the step-by-step protocol that matches your selection.

②

Select an ailment category

Once you have determined your goal, you need to determine which ailment category you'd like to use. Do you want to address the issue by:

LOCATION → WHERE?

BODY SYSTEM → WHICH ONE?

CHAKRA → WHICH ONE?

PRELIMINARY STEPS

There are four preparatory steps you need to complete before beginning a Reiki session. Here, we tell you what these steps are—the following pages will explain each of these steps in detail.

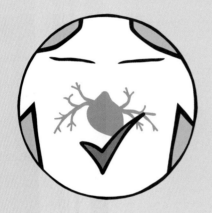

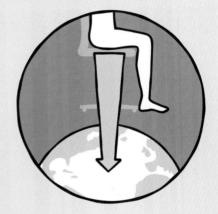

1

Setting your Intention

PAGES 20-21

2

Centering and Grounding

PAGES 22-25

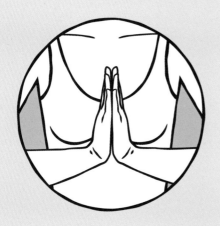

3

Reciting the Reiki Prayer

PAGE 26

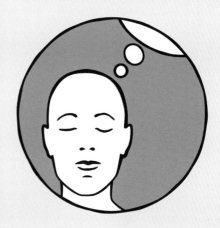

4

Reciting Reiki Affirmations

PAGE 27

1 SETTING YOUR INTENTION

Intention is a powerful tool for creating a powerful session.

Intention of the sender

As a sender of subtle energy, it is critical that your intention is pure and unattached. Results are not your concern. The session is for the receiver, and you are merely a conduit through which the work can unfold.

Your job is to stay out of the way and remain focused on your intention to facilitate the receiver's own body's ability to heal itself. You are not in a position to know what, if anything, is needed, or if anything should occur.

Intention of the receiver

If someone has agreed that you may work on them, they are at the very least willing to try to receive the work. It is not appropriate to force someone to do a session or to do the work without their permission. Clearly, you are not in control of the intentions of the receiver. However, you can help them to identify or clarify their intention for the session.

You can show the receiver some of the affirmations included in this book, or any others that you feel are appropriate, and invite him or her to recite the affirmations aloud before the session. You can also ask questions that will encourage the receiver to consider what they would like to achieve from the session. For example, you might ask:

WHAT WOULD YOU LIKE TO
GET OUT OF THE SESSION?

*

HOW WOULD YOU LIKE TO FEEL
AT THE END OF THE SESSION?

*

DO YOU HAVE ANY
DISCOMFORT IN YOUR BODY?

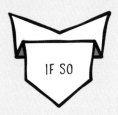

IF SO

CAN YOU DESCRIBE IT?

FOLLOWED
BY

DOES IT HAVE COLOR, TEXTURE,
TEMPERATURE, OR SOUND?

*

IF THE DISCOMFORT IS GONE AT THE END OF THE
SESSION, WHAT WOULD IT " LOOK" LIKE THEN?

2 CENTERING & GROUNDING

Regardless of which protocol you intend to use, follow the personal preparation steps below—before your receiver has arrived—for centering yourself:

STEP 1 CENTER YOURSELF (BEFORE YOUR RECEIVER HAS ARRIVED)

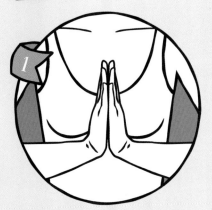

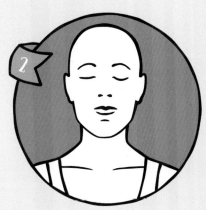

Sit upright in a comfortable chair and with both feet flat on the floor. Place your hands in Prayer Pose, with the heels of your palms and fingertips pressing against each other and the sides of your thumbs pressing against your chest.

Close your eyes, and gently press your tongue on the roof of your mouth, just behind your front teeth.

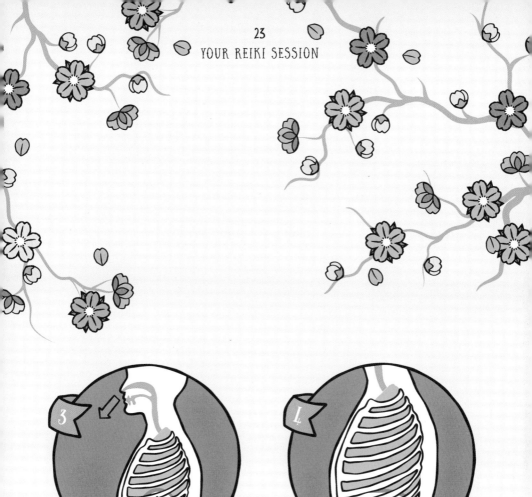

Perform long, deep breathing by slowly inhaling for eight seconds through your nose, allowing your belly to expand just below the navel, and then gently exhaling through your nose for another eight seconds. Do this for three cycles (48 seconds).

Repeat the long, deep breathing cycle, this time holding your breath for five seconds between the inhale and the exhale and for five seconds at the end of the exhale. Do this for three cycles (78 seconds). Continue breathing comfortably at your own pace.

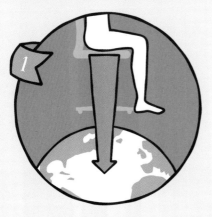

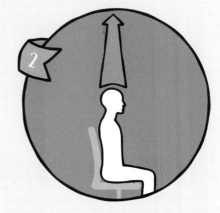

With your eyes closed, ground yourself and the space by visualizing a connection from your tailbone to the center of the earth.

Simultaneously visualize a connection from the top of your head to the sky above you. This may create a perceptible "tension," pulling gently in each direction.

BALANCING THE TENSION

If you are feeling low energy/ lethargic, focus more on the connection to the sky. Conversely, if you are feeling high energy/anxious, focus more on the connection to the center of the earth. This will help balance the tension of grounding and connecting.

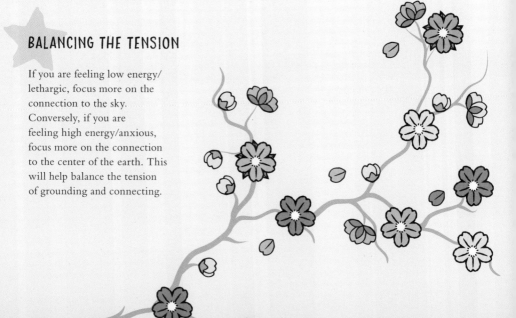

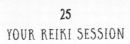
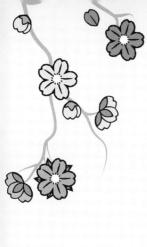
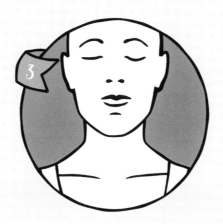

Now, set an intention for yourself/your friend or family member. "Trust and allow" is a great mantra for setting your intention. Trust that the process will work in the highest interests of the sender and receiver, and allow the session to unfold without making it mean anything. Some examples of mantras are:

I fill the space with golden-light energy that is calming and nurturing.

❋

I trust that the Universal Life Energy will provide healing and vitalizing assistance to the receiver where it is needed.

❋

I allow the Universal Life Energy to move with ease through me to the receiver with no attachment to any particular result or outcome.

3 RECITING THE REIKI PRAYER

Just for today...

*

I let go of anger

*

I let go of worry

*

I am grateful

*

I work on myself

*

I am kind to all living things

4. RECITING REIKI AFFIRMATIONS

I am healing

WORRY IS GONE. I AM REMEMBERING TO SMILE.

I am peace

ANGER IS GONE. I AM REMEMBERING TO LAUGH.

I am abundance

SCARCITY IS GONE. I AM REMEMBERING TO
WORK HONESTLY AND BE GENEROUS.

I am joy

SORROW IS GONE. I AM REMEMBERING TO REJOICE
AND BE THANKFUL FOR MY MANY BLESSINGS.

I am love

FEAR IS GONE. I AM REMEMBERING TO BE KIND
TO MY NEIGHBOR AND ALL LIVING THINGS.

I am life

SEPARATION IS GONE. I AM REMEMBERING TO BE HAPPY.

DOING YOUR SESSION

Now you're fully prepared, you will need to make sure that the space in which you will hold the session is appropriately set up and that you prepare your receiver (if relevant).

THE SPACE

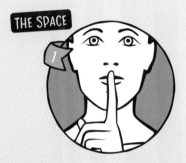

Select a quiet space, where you will have minimum or no interruption.

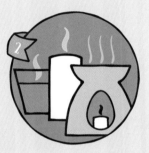

If you can, and if you want to, light some candles and burn some incense, or use an essential oil diffuser to create a calm and relaxing atmosphere.

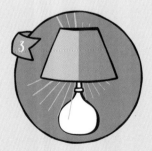

Play quiet instrumental music and dim the lighting in the room.

NOTE: SITTING COMFORTABLY

- The session can be done sitting upright in a chair, but make adjustments to comfortably do the hand positions described in the protocols. It is completely effective to approximate the placement of the hand positions.
- If you are doing a self-help session, it can be done sitting comfortably in a chair with your feet flat on the floor.

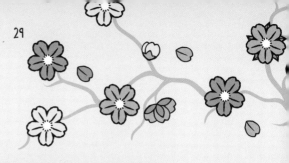

RECEIVER PREPARATION

IF YOU ARE DOING A SELF-HELP SESSION, SKIP THE RECEIVER PREPARATION BELOW AND GO DIRECTLY TO THE REIKI PRAYER AND AFFIRMATIONS.

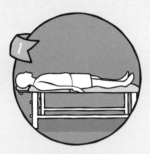

Have a massage table set up for the receiver. Family-help sessions are best done with the receiver lying on his or her back on a massage table. If you do not have a table, you can have the receiver sit in a reclining lounge chair or lay on a comfortable sofa. Have a blanket ready in case the receiver gets chilly.

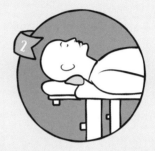

Be sure to ask the receiver to let you know if he or she is uncomfortable at any point in the session. Nothing done in the session should be painful. Make sure that your receiver has neck and lower back support if needed, such as a neck pillow or a bolster for the back of the knees.

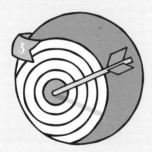

Remind the receiver of the goal of the session and ask if there is a particular intention. (Ideally, you will have already spoken to the receiver and will know what type of session you will be doing ahead of time.)

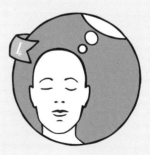

Invoke the Reiki Prayer by reciting it silently to yourself.

The best things in life are nearest: breath in your nostrils, light in your eyes, flowers at your feet, duties at your hand, the path of right just before you.

Then do not grasp at the stars, but do life's plain, common work as it comes, certain that daily duties and daily bread are the sweetest things in life.

Robert Louis Stevenson

2
TRADITIONAL HAND POSITIONS

PROTOCOL FOR OVERALL WELL-BEING OF YOURSELF

IN ADDITION TO FACILITATING THE BODY'S OWN SELF—HEALING, REIKI AND SUBTLE ENERGY WORK CAN ALSO BE USED TO PROMOTE AND MAINTAIN WELLNESS.

YOU DON'T NEED TO BE SICK TO BENEFIT FROM ENERGY WORK! IF THERE IS A SIMPLE WAY TO HELP YOU STAY HEALTHY, WHY NOT INCLUDE IT AS A PART OF YOUR COMMITMENT TO YOUR OWN WELLNESS?

THE HUMAN BODY IS CONSTANTLY PERFORMING HOUSEKEEPING TASKS. WITHIN EACH CELL OF EVERY TISSUE OF EVERY ORGAN, METABOLIC PROCESSES ARE OCCURRING. THESE PROCESSES UTILIZE NUTRIENTS TO PRODUCE SUBSTANCES NEEDED FOR A HEALTHY BODY, BUT THEY ALSO RESULT IN A VARIETY OF WASTE BYPRODUCTS THAT ARE EFFICIENTLY ELIMINATED BY THE BODY.

AS A NORMAL PART OF THIS METABOLIC PROCESS SOME OF THE CELLS MAY MALFUNCTION, AND UNDER IDEAL CIRCUMSTANCES THE BODY WILL RECOGNIZE THE PROBLEM CELLS AND ACTIVELY SEEK THEM OUT TO BE DESTROYED AND ELIMINATED FROM THE BODY. ANYTHING THAT HELPS THE BODY PERFORM THIS VITAL FUNCTION IS BENEFICIAL TO OVERALL WELL-BEING. REIKI AND SUBTLE ENERGY WORK MAY ASSIST THE HOUSEKEEPING PROCESS BY PROVIDING AN EXTERNAL SOURCE OF ENERGY TO THE SYSTEM, ALONG WITH AN INTENTION FOR WELL-BEING.

REIKI AND SUBTLE ENERGY WORK ARE SIMPLE AND EASY TO USE, AND WELL WORTH INCLUDING IN YOUR REGULAR WELLNESS REGIMEN. THEY JUST MIGHT MAKE YOUR FEELING OF OVERALL WELL-BEING GO FROM GOOD TO GREAT!

Self Help **H1: EYES**

① **Close your eyes and cup your hands.**

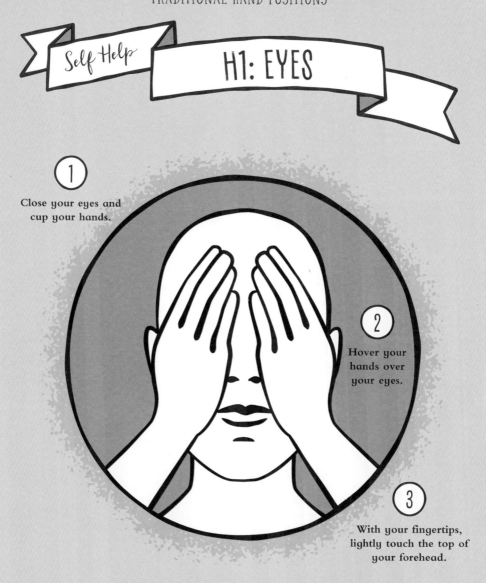

② **Hover your hands over your eyes.**

③ **With your fingertips, lightly touch the top of your forehead.**

Begin long and deep breathing, and visualize the Reiki Universal Life Energy flowing from the **palms of your hands** toward your **eyes**. Using your mind's eye, "see" the energy moving into the **center of your head** through the **eyes** and **sinuses**, into the **center of your brain**, and surrounding your **pituitary** and **pineal glands** and your **hypothalamus**.

HEAD

H2: TEMPLES

Self Help

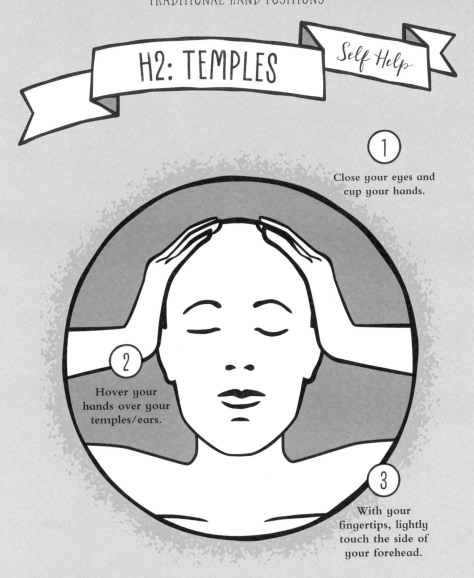

1

Close your eyes and cup your hands.

2

Hover your hands over your temples/ears.

3

With your fingertips, lightly touch the side of your forehead.

Begin long and deep breathing, and visualize the Reiki Universal Life Energy flowing from the **palms of your hands** toward your **temples**. Using your mind's eye, "see" the energy moving into the **center of your head**, through your **inner ear**, **eyes**, and **optic nerves**, and the **frontal lobe of the brain**.

HEAD

Self Help

H3: SKULL

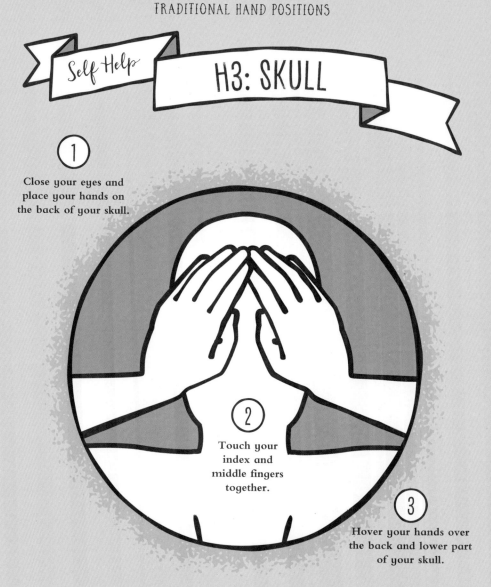

① Close your eyes and place your hands on the back of your skull.

② Touch your index and middle fingers together.

③ Hover your hands over the back and lower part of your skull.

Begin long and deep breathing, and visualize the Reiki Universal Life Energy flowing from the **palms of your hands** toward the **front of your skull.** Using your mind's eye, "see" the energy moving into the **center of your head** through the **cerebellum** and **brain stem** at the base of your skull.

HEAD

H4: THROAT

Self Help

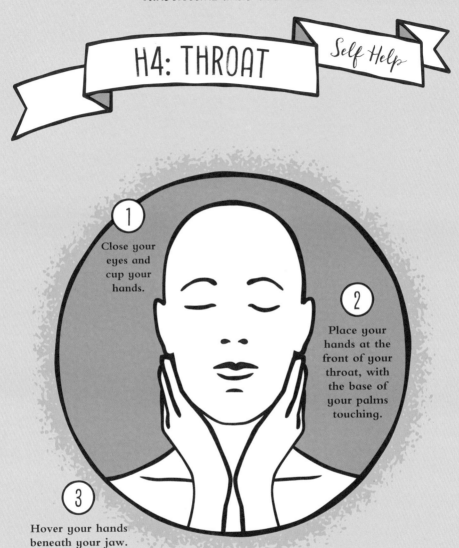

1 Close your eyes and cup your hands.

2 Place your hands at the front of your throat, with the base of your palms touching.

3 Hover your hands beneath your jaw.

Begin long and deep breathing, and visualize the Reiki Universal Life Energy flowing from the **palms of your hands** toward your **throat**. Using your mind's eye, "see" the energy moving from your **throat** through and around the **back of your neck**.

HEAD

Self Help

F1: HEART

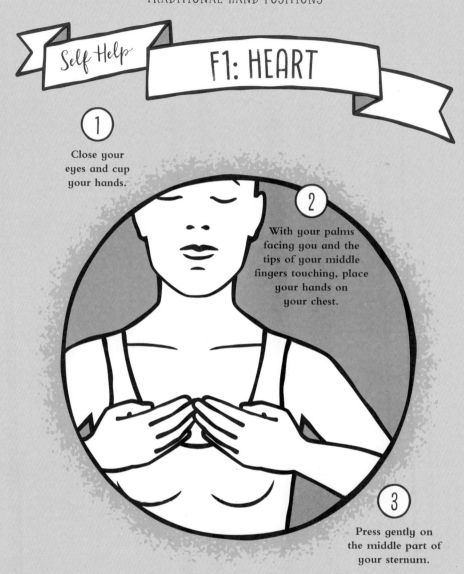

1 Close your eyes and cup your hands.

2 With your palms facing you and the tips of your middle fingers touching, place your hands on your chest.

3 Press gently on the middle part of your sternum.

Begin long and deep breathing, and visualize the Reiki Universal Life Energy flowing from the **palms of your hands** toward your **heart**. Using your mind's eye, "see" the energy moving from the **front of your chest**, through your **lungs** and **heart**, and around toward your **back**.

FRONT

F2: SOLAR PLEXUS

Self Help

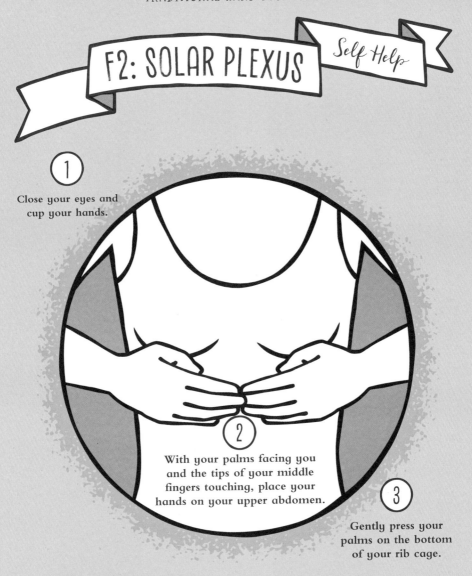

1 Close your eyes and cup your hands.

2 With your palms facing you and the tips of your middle fingers touching, place your hands on your upper abdomen.

3 Gently press your palms on the bottom of your rib cage.

Begin long and deep breathing, and visualize the Reiki Universal Life Energy flowing from the **palms of your hands** toward your **solar plexus**, just below the diaphragm. Using your mind's eye, "see" the energy moving from the front of your **rib cage** through your **upper abdomen**, surrounding your **major organs—stomach, pancreas, liver, gallbladder, kidneys,** and **spleen.**

FRONT

Self Help — F3: NAVEL

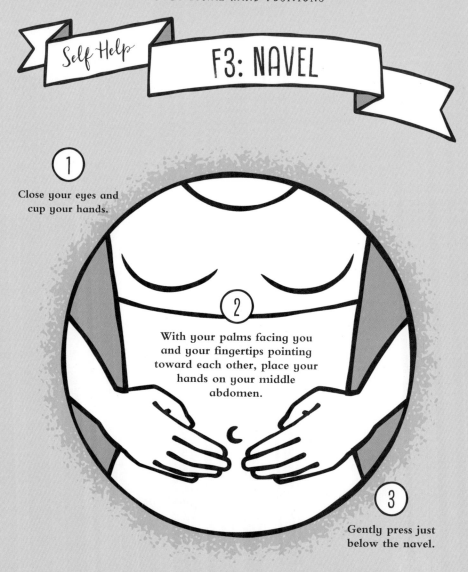

1 Close your eyes and cup your hands.

2 With your palms facing you and your fingertips pointing toward each other, place your hands on your middle abdomen.

3 Gently press just below the navel.

Begin long and deep breathing, and visualize the Reiki Universal Life Energy flowing from the **palms of your hands** toward your **navel**. Using your mind's eye, "see" the energy moving from your **navel** into your **mid-abdomen**, surrounding your **large** and **small intestines, ureters, greater** and **lesser omentum**, and **mesentery**.

FRONT

F4: GROIN

Self Help

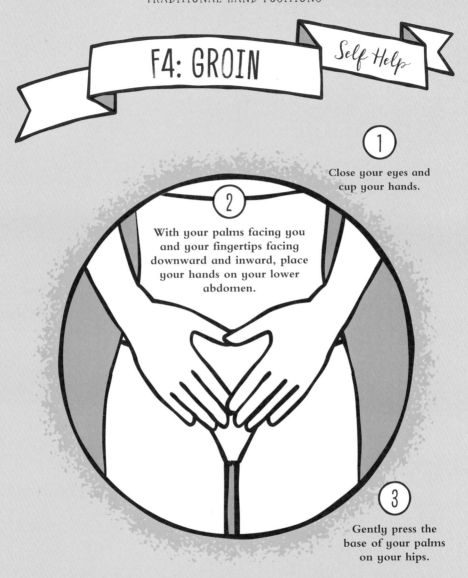

1

Close your eyes and cup your hands.

2

With your palms facing you and your fingertips facing downward and inward, place your hands on your lower abdomen.

3

Gently press the base of your palms on your hips.

Begin long and deep breathing, and visualize the Reiki Universal Life Energy flowing from the **palms of your hands** toward your **groin**. Using your mind's eye, "see" the energy moving from the **front of your pelvis** through your **reproductive organs, appendix, urinary bladder, sigmoid colon, rectum**, and **anus**.

FRONT

Self Help

B1: SHOULDERS

①

Close your eyes and
cup your hands.

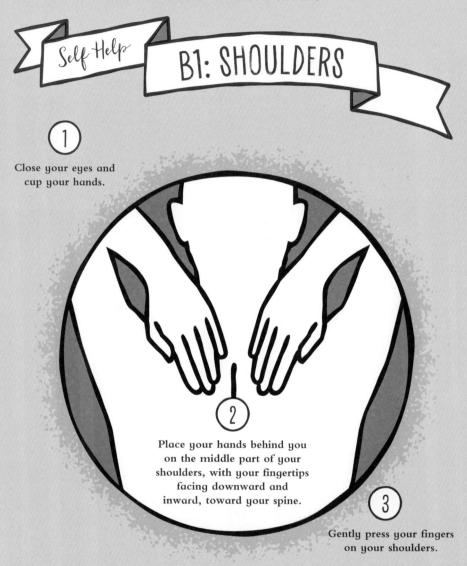

②

Place your hands behind you
on the middle part of your
shoulders, with your fingertips
facing downward and
inward, toward your spine.

③

Gently press your fingers
on your shoulders.

Begin long and deep breathing, and visualize the Reiki Universal Life Energy
flowing from the **palms of your hands** toward your **shoulders**. Using your
mind's eye, "see" the energy moving across the top of your **shoulders** and down
your **spine** and **ribs** through your **lungs** and **heart**.

BACK

B2: RIBS

Self Help

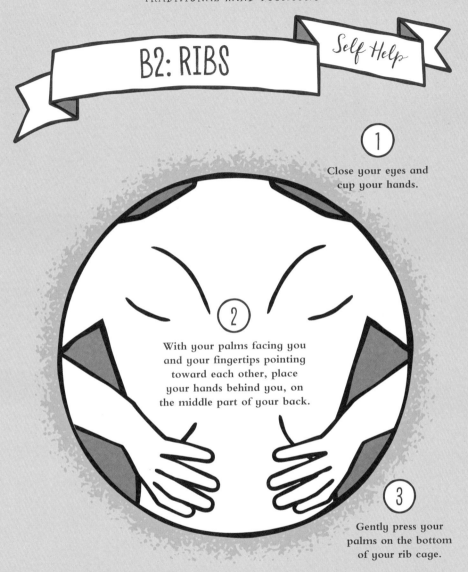

1

Close your eyes and cup your hands.

2

With your palms facing you and your fingertips pointing toward each other, place your hands behind you, on the middle part of your back.

3

Gently press your palms on the bottom of your rib cage.

Begin long and deep breathing, and visualize the Reiki Universal Life Energy flowing from the **palms of your hands** toward your **middle back**. Using your mind's eye, "see" the energy moving from your **ribs**, through your **upper abdomen**, and surrounding your **major organs— stomach, pancreas, liver, gallbladder, kidneys**, and **spleen**.

BACK

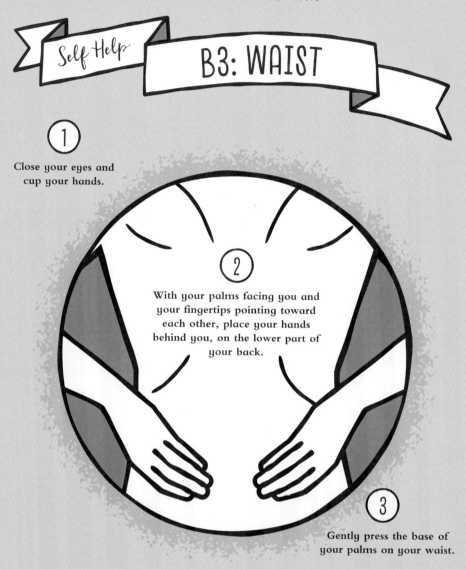

Self Help

B3: WAIST

1 Close your eyes and cup your hands.

2 With your palms facing you and your fingertips pointing toward each other, place your hands behind you, on the lower part of your back.

3 Gently press the base of your palms on your waist.

Begin long and deep breathing, and visualize the Reiki Universal Life Energy flowing from the **palms of your hands** toward your **waist**. Using your mind's eye, "see" the energy moving from your **lower back** into your **mid-abdomen**, surrounding your **large** and **small intestines, ureters, greater** and **lesser omentum**, and **mesentery**.

BACK

B4: COCCYX

Self Help

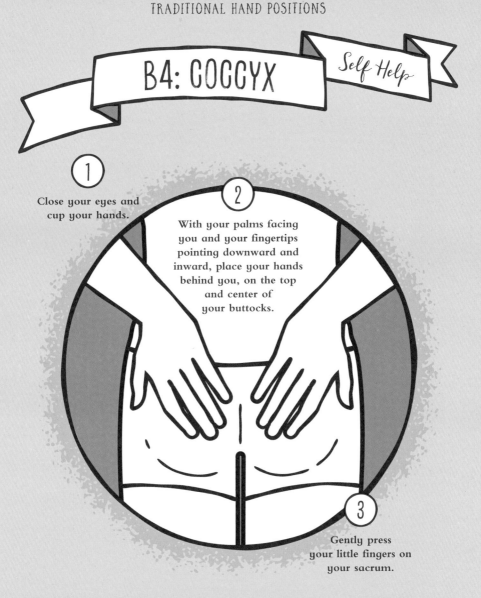

1 Close your eyes and cup your hands.

2 With your palms facing you and your fingertips pointing downward and inward, place your hands behind you, on the top and center of your buttocks.

3 Gently press your little fingers on your sacrum.

Begin long and deep breathing, and visualize the Reiki Universal Life Energy flowing from the **palms of your hands** toward your **sacrum** and **coccyx**. Using your mind's eye, "see" the energy moving from the **back of your pelvis** through your **reproductive organs, appendix, urinary bladder, sigmoid colon, rectum**, and **anus**.

BACK

Self Help

L1: KNEE

①
Close your eyes and
cup your hands.

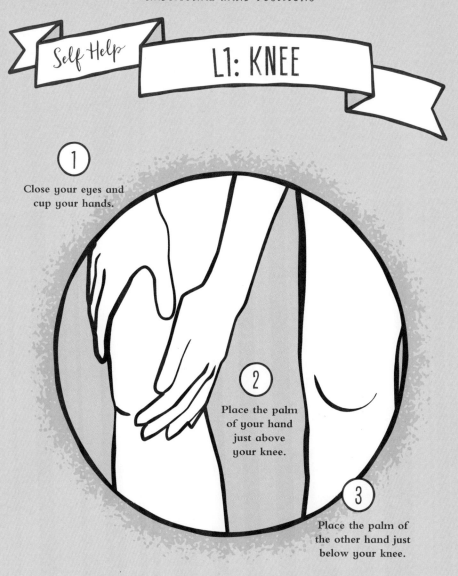

②
Place the palm
of your hand
just above
your knee.

③
Place the palm of
the other hand just
below your knee.

Begin long and deep breathing, and visualize the Reiki Universal Life Energy flowing from the **palms of your hands**. Using your mind's eye, "see" the energy moving from the top of your **kneecap**, up and around the **leg** toward your **hip**, and down and around the **shin** toward your **foot**. (Switch hand position to your other leg and repeat L1 technique.)

LEGS/FEET

L2: ANKLE

Self Help

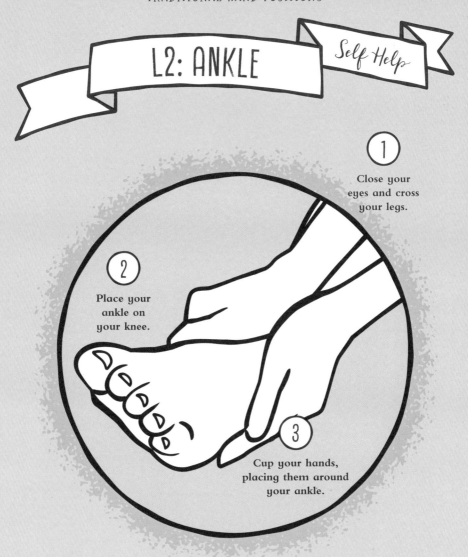

1 Close your eyes and cross your legs.

2 Place your ankle on your knee.

3 Cup your hands, placing them around your ankle.

Begin long and deep breathing, and visualize the Reiki Universal Life Energy flowing from the **palms of your hands**. Using your mind's eye, "see" the energy moving through and around your **ankle** and your **heel**. (Switch hand position to your other leg and repeat L2 technique.)

LEGS/FEET

Self Help

L3: SOLE

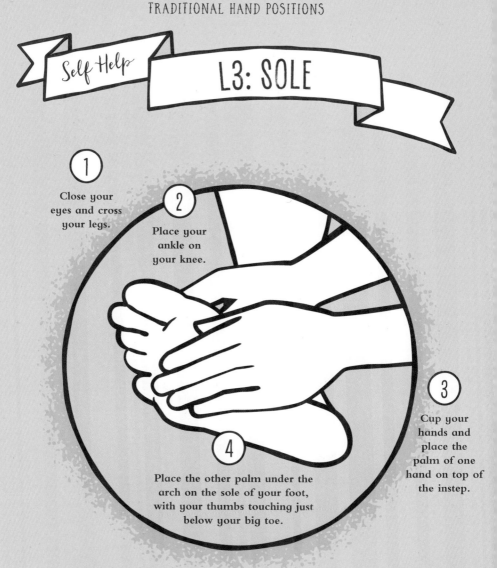

1 Close your eyes and cross your legs.

2 Place your ankle on your knee.

3 Cup your hands and place the palm of one hand on top of the instep.

4 Place the other palm under the arch on the sole of your foot, with your thumbs touching just below your big toe.

Begin long and deep breathing, and visualize the Reiki Universal Life Energy flowing from the **palms of your hands**. Using your mind's eye, "see" the energy moving through and around your **foot** toward your **toes**. (Switch hand position to your other leg and repeat L3 technique.)

H1: EYES

Family Help

① Cup your hands, with the sides of your thumbs touching and your fingers facing away from you.

② Gently place the base of your palms on the top of the forehead.

③ Hover over the eyes and cheeks.

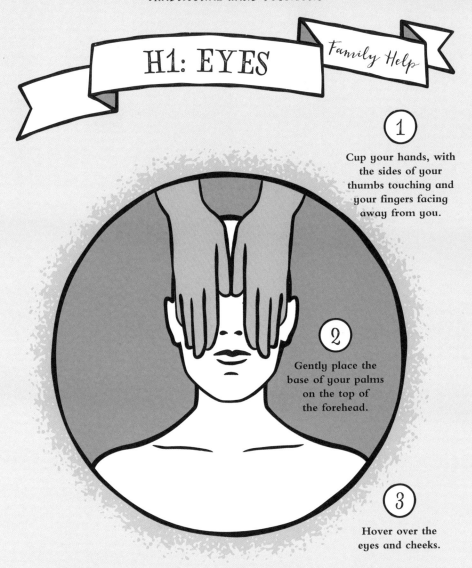

Begin long and deep breathing, and begin to visualize the Reiki Universal Life Energy flowing from the **palms of your hands** toward the **eyes**. Using your mind's eye, "see" the energy moving into the **center of the head**, through the **eyes** and **sinuses**, into the **center of the brain**, and surrounding the **pituitary** and **pineal glands** and the **hypothalamus**.

HEAD

Family Help

H2: TEMPLES

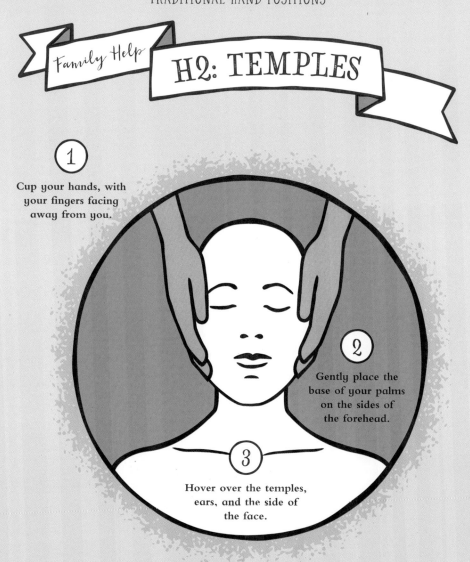

1 Cup your hands, with your fingers facing away from you.

2 Gently place the base of your palms on the sides of the forehead.

3 Hover over the temples, ears, and the side of the face.

Begin long and deep breathing, and visualize the Reiki Universal Life Energy flowing from the **palms of your hands** toward the **temples**. Using your mind's eye, "see" the energy moving into the **center of the head**, through the **inner ear, eyes, optic nerves**, and muscles of the **jaw**.

HEAD

H3: SKULL

Family Help

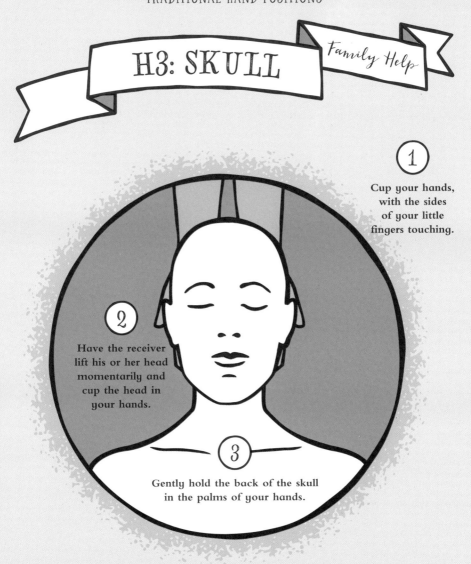

1
Cup your hands, with the sides of your little fingers touching.

2
Have the receiver lift his or her head momentarily and cup the head in your hands.

3
Gently hold the back of the skull in the palms of your hands.

Begin long and deep breathing, and visualize the Reiki Universal Life Energy flowing from the **palms of your hands** toward the **front of the skull**. Using your mind's eye, "see" the energy moving into the **center of the head** through the **cerebellum** and **brain stem** at the base of skull.

HEAD

Family Help

H4: THROAT

1

Cup your hands, with your index and middle fingers touching.

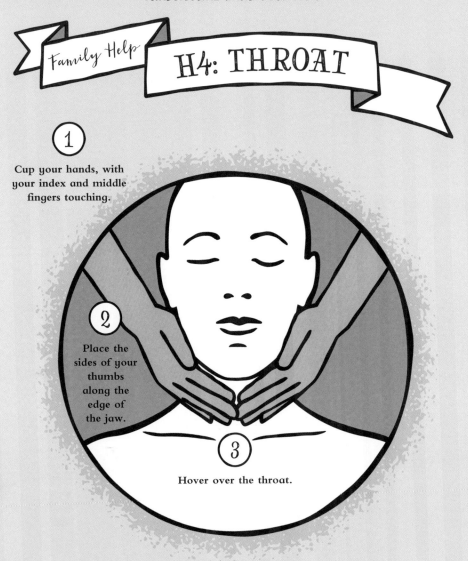

2

Place the sides of your thumbs along the edge of the jaw.

3

Hover over the throat.

Begin long and deep breathing, and visualize the Reiki Universal Life Energy flowing from the **palms of your hands** toward the **throat**. Using your mind's eye, "see" the energy moving from the **throat** through and around the **back of the neck**.

HEAD

F1: HEART

Family Help

1

Cup your hands and place them perpendicular to each other.

2

Face your palms downward, with the fingertips of one hand facing the feet and the fingertips of the other facing away from you.

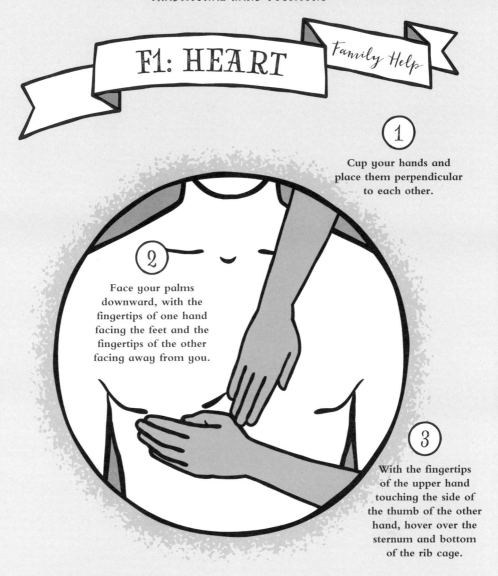

3

With the fingertips of the upper hand touching the side of the thumb of the other hand, hover over the sternum and bottom of the rib cage.

Begin long and deep breathing, and visualize the Reiki Universal Life Energy flowing from the **palms of your hands** toward the **heart**. Using your mind's eye, "see" the energy moving from the **front of the chest**, through the **lungs** and **heart**, and around toward the **back**.

FRONT

Family Help

F2: SOLAR PLEXUS

1 Cup your hands and place them in tandem, with your fingertips facing away from you.

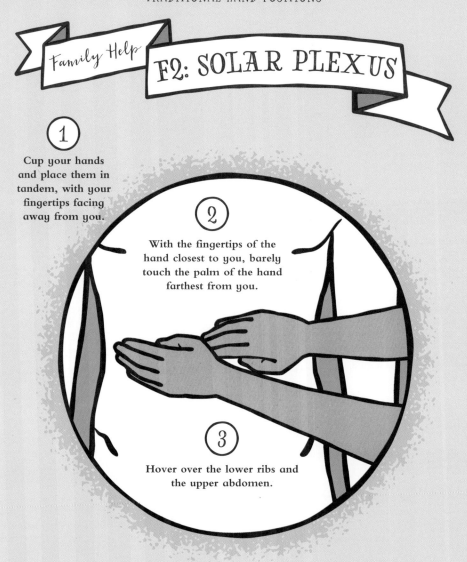

2 With the fingertips of the hand closest to you, barely touch the palm of the hand farthest from you.

3 Hover over the lower ribs and the upper abdomen.

Begin long and deep breathing, and visualize the Reiki Universal Life Energy flowing from the **palms of your hands** toward the **solar plexus**. Using your mind's eye, "see" the energy moving from the **front of the rib cage**, through the **upper abdomen**, and surrounding the **major organs—stomach, pancreas, liver, gallbladder, kidneys,** and **spleen**.

FRONT

F3: NAVEL

Family Help

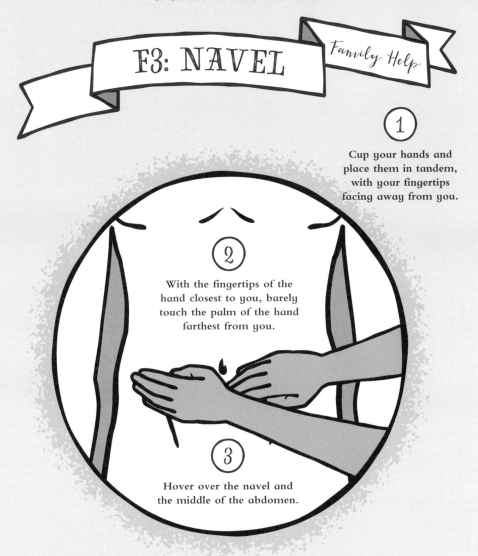

1

Cup your hands and place them in tandem, with your fingertips facing away from you.

2

With the fingertips of the hand closest to you, barely touch the palm of the hand farthest from you.

3

Hover over the navel and the middle of the abdomen.

Begin long and deep breathing, and visualize the Reiki Universal Life Energy flowing from the **palms of your hands** toward the **navel**. Using your mind's eye, "see" the energy moving from the **navel** into the **mid-abdomen**, surrounding the **large** and **small intestines, ureters, greater** and **lesser omentum**, and **mesentery**.

FRONT

Family Help

F4: GROIN

1

Cup your hands and place them in tandem, with your fingertips facing away from you.

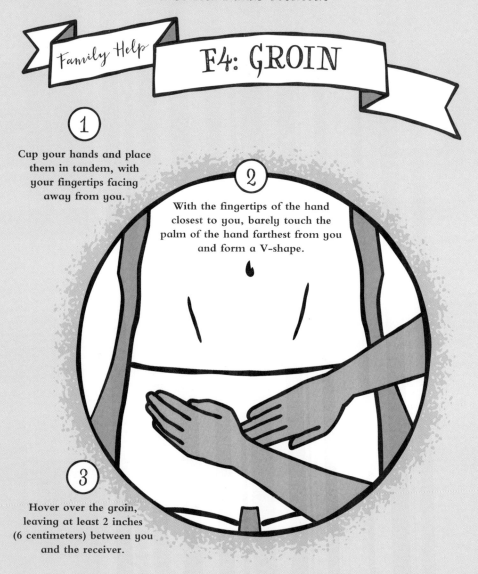

2

With the fingertips of the hand closest to you, barely touch the palm of the hand farthest from you and form a V-shape.

3

Hover over the groin, leaving at least 2 inches (6 centimeters) between you and the receiver.

Begin long and deep breathing, and visualize the Reiki Universal Life Energy flowing from the **palms of your hands** toward the **groin**. Using your mind's eye, "see" the energy moving from the **front of the pelvis** through the **reproductive organs, appendix, urinary bladder, sigmoid colon, rectum,** and **anus**.

FRONT

B1: SHOULDERS

Family Help

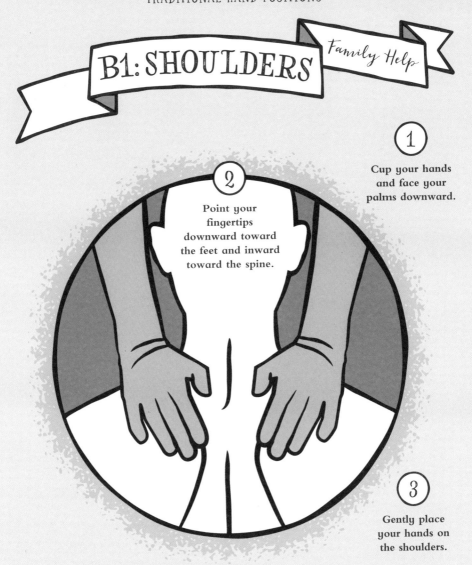

1
Cup your hands and face your palms downward.

2
Point your fingertips downward toward the feet and inward toward the spine.

3
Gently place your hands on the shoulders.

Begin long and deep breathing, and visualize the Reiki Universal Life Energy flowing from the **palms of your hands** toward the **shoulders**. Using your mind's eye, "see" the energy moving across the **top of the shoulders** and down the **spine** and **ribs**.

BACK

Family Help

B2: RIBS

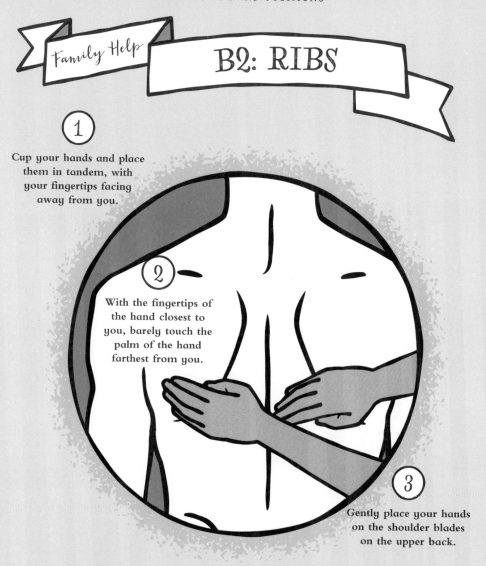

1

Cup your hands and place them in tandem, with your fingertips facing away from you.

2

With the fingertips of the hand closest to you, barely touch the palm of the hand farthest from you.

3

Gently place your hands on the shoulder blades on the upper back.

Begin long and deep breathing, and visualize the Reiki Universal Life Energy flowing from the **palms of your hands** toward the **middle back**. Using your mind's eye, "see" the energy moving from the **back of the chest**, through the **lungs** and **heart**, and around toward the **front of the chest**.

BACK

B3: WAIST

Family Help

① Cup your hands and place them in tandem, with your fingertips facing away from you.

② With the fingertips of the hand closest to you, barely touch the palm of the hand farthest from you.

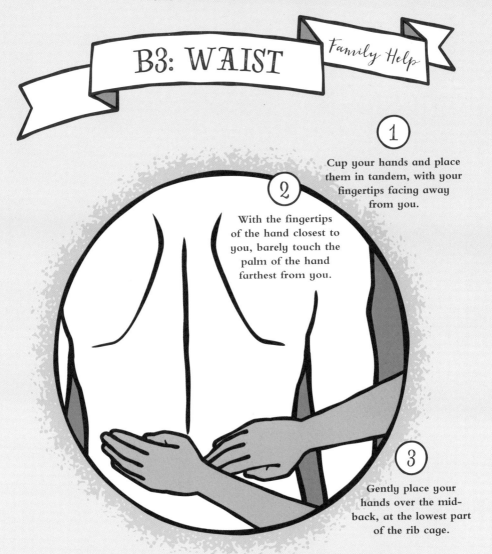

③ Gently place your hands over the mid-back, at the lowest part of the rib cage.

Begin long and deep breathing, and visualize the Reiki Universal Life Energy flowing from the **palms of your hands** toward the **waist**. Using your mind's eye, "see" the energy moving from the **ribs**, through the **upper abdomen**, and surrounding the **major organs—stomach, pancreas, liver, gallbladder, kidneys,** and **spleen**.

BACK

Family Help

B4: COCCYX

1

Cup your hands and place them in tandem, with your fingertips facing away from you.

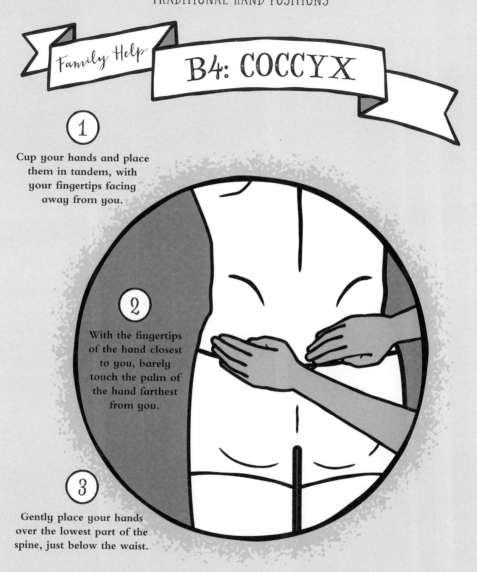

2

With the fingertips of the hand closest to you, barely touch the palm of the hand farthest from you.

3

Gently place your hands over the lowest part of the spine, just below the waist.

Begin long and deep breathing, and visualize the Reiki Universal Life Energy flowing from the **palms of your hands** toward the **sacrum** and **coccyx**. Using your mind's eye, "see" the energy moving from the **upper buttocks** through the **reproductive organs, appendix, urinary bladder, sigmoid colon, rectum,** and **anus**.

BACK

L1: KNEE

Family Help

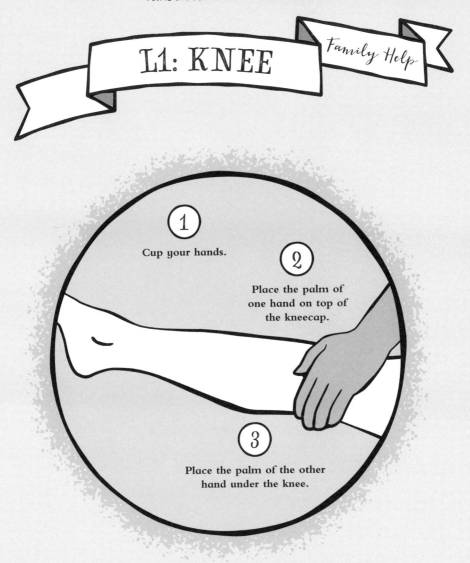

1 Cup your hands.

2 Place the palm of one hand on top of the kneecap.

3 Place the palm of the other hand under the knee.

Begin long and deep breathing, and visualize the Reiki Universal Life Energy flowing from the **palms of your hands**. Using your mind's eye, "see" the energy moving from the **top of the kneecap**, up and around the **leg** toward the **hip**, and down and around the **shin** toward the **foot**. (Switch hand position to the other leg and repeat L1 technique.)

LEGS/FEET

Family Help

L2: ANKLE

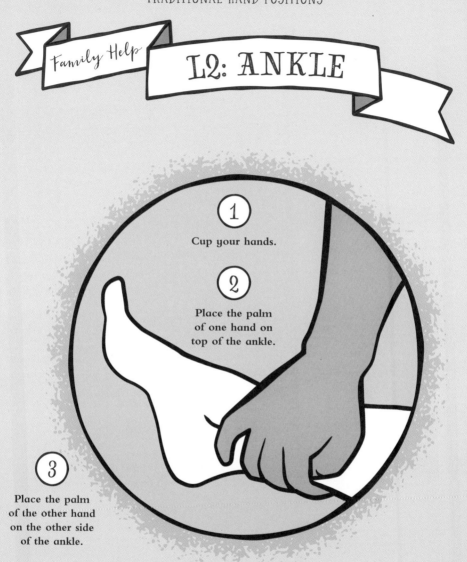

1 Cup your hands.

2 Place the palm of one hand on top of the ankle.

3 Place the palm of the other hand on the other side of the ankle.

Begin long and deep breathing, and visualize the Reiki Universal Life Energy flowing from the **palms of your hands**. Using your mind's eye, "see" the energy moving through and around the **ankle** and the **heel**. (Switch hand position to the other leg and repeat L2 technique.)

LEGS/FEET

L3: SOLE

Family Help

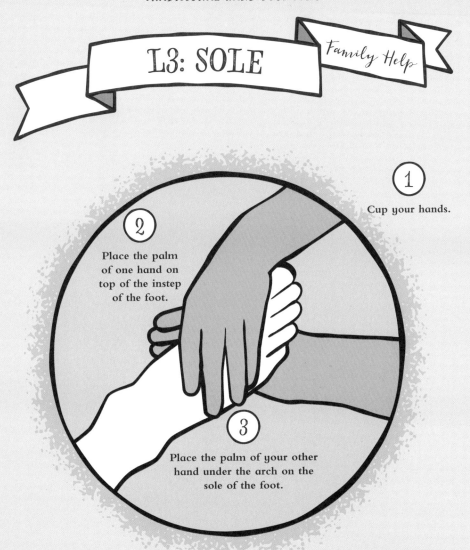

① Cup your hands.

② Place the palm of one hand on top of the instep of the foot.

③ Place the palm of your other hand under the arch on the sole of the foot.

Begin long and deep breathing, and visualize the Reiki Universal Life Energy flowing from the **palms of your hands**. Using your mind's eye, "see" the energy moving through and around the **foot** toward the **toes**. (Switch hand position to the other leg and repeat L3 technique.)

LEGS/FEET

To see a world in a grain of sand

And a heaven in a wild flower.

Hold infinity in the palm of your hand

And eternity in an hour.

William Blake

3 AILMENT CATEGORIES

FOR SPECIFIC SYMPTOMS

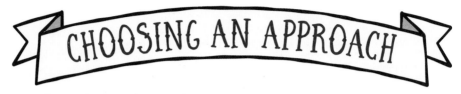

CHOOSING AN APPROACH

Depending on the specific symptom or ailment, you will need to choose a treatment. First, determine which ailment category type (by physical location, body system, or chakra) you think is most appropriate. You can then learn a specific protocol to achieve your goal. This article will help you make up your mind.

PHYSICAL LOCATION

HEAD & NECK/CHEST/UPPER ABDOMEN/PELVIS/LEGS & FEET

Sometimes, there is discomfort or disease in a particular part of the body without the cause or source being known. One of the amazing properties of Reiki energy is that it goes where it is needed most, without having to know why an issue exists. By following a protocol that uses hand positions associated with particular locations in the body, you can begin to address some of these issues.

BODY SYSTEMS

Internal processes operate to keep the conditions in your body within tight limits, allowing metabolic chemical reactions to proceed. Homeostatic processes act at the level of the cell, the tissue, and the organ, as well as for the organism as a whole.

By following a protocol that uses hand positions associated with particular imbalances in one or more of these systems, you may begin to address some of the issues caused by stress or injuries acquired in your daily life.

IMMUNE SYSTEM: Thymus and bone marrow, spleen, tonsils, lymph vessels, lymph nodes, adenoids, skin, and liver

CIRCULATORY SYSTEM: Heart and blood vessels

GASTROINTESTINAL SYSTEM: Stomach, small and large intestines, pancreas, liver, gallbladder

RESPIRATORY SYSTEM: Throat, lungs

ENDOCRINE SYSTEM: Pituitary, pineal, thyroid, adrenals, gonads

THE CHAKRAS

The chakras are centers in your body associated with physical organs or glands through which energy spins and flows. Blocked energy in any of our seven chakras can sometimes lead to illness, so it is important to understand what each chakra represents and what you can do to encourage this energy to flow freely. By following a protocol that uses hand positions associated with particular imbalances in one or more of these chakras, you may begin to ensure that your chakras stay open, aligned, and fluid.

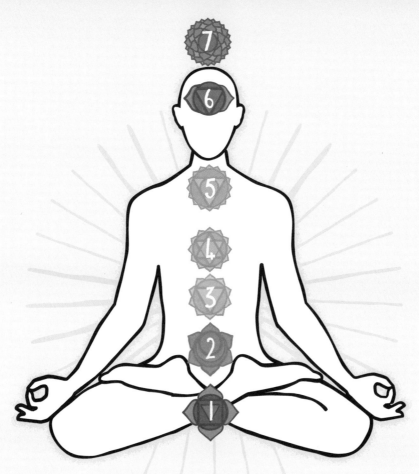

1) **ROOT CHAKRA**
Base of the spine
• Security,
vulnerability
• Trust

2) **SACRAL CHAKRA**
Just below navel
• Passion,
inspiration,
procreation
• Sexuality,
creativity

3) **SOLAR PLEXUS
CHAKRA**
Stomach
• Core power,
fortitude
• Wisdom, power

4) **HEART CHAKRA**
Center of the chest
• Compassion,
empathy
• Love, healing

5) **THROAT CHAKRA**
Base of the throat
• Self-expression,
voice
• Communication

6) **THIRD EYE
CHAKRA**
Forehead, just
above and between
the eyes
• Intuition, inner
vision
• Awareness

7) **CROWN CHAKRA**
Top of the head
• Connection to
higher self
• Spirituality

AILMENTS BY PHYSICAL LOCATION

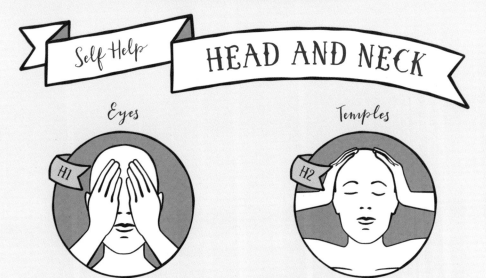

Self Help

HEAD AND NECK

Eyes

H1

Close your eyes and cup your hands. Hover your hands over your **eyes**. With your fingertips, lightly touch the **top of your forehead**.

Temples

H2

Close your eyes and cup your hands. Hover your hands over your **temples/ears**. With your fingertips, lightly touch the **side of your forehead**.

Skull

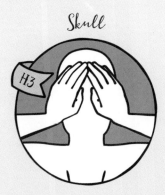

H3

Close your eyes and place your hands on the **back of your skull**. Touch your index and middle fingers together. Hover your hands over the **back and lower part of your skull**.

Throat

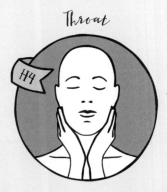

H4

Close your eyes and cup your hands. Place your hands at the **front of your throat**, with the base of your palms touching. Hover beneath your **jaw**.

CHEST

Self Help

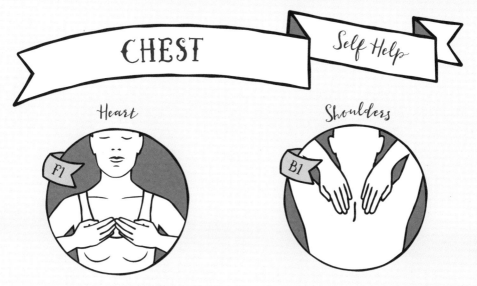

Heart

Close your eyes and cup your hands. With your palms facing you and the tips of your middle fingers touching, place your hands on your **chest**. Press gently on the middle part of your **sternum**.

Shoulders

Close your eyes and cup your hands. Place your hands behind you on the middle part of your **shoulders,** with your fingertips facing downward and inward, toward your **spine**. Gently press your fingers on your **shoulders**.

Ribs

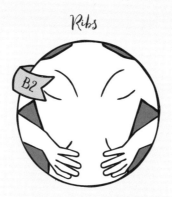

Close your eyes and cup your hands. With your palms facing you and your fingertips pointing toward each other, place your hands behind you, on the **middle part of your back**. Gently press your palms on the **bottom of your rib cage**.

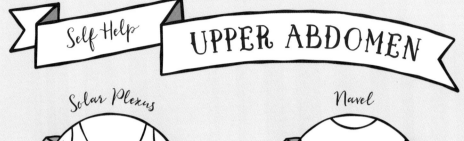

Self Help — UPPER ABDOMEN

Solar Plexus

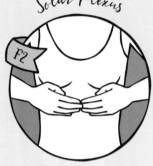

Close your eyes and cup your hands. With your palms facing you and the tips of your middle fingers touching, place your hands on your **upper abdomen**. Gently press your palms on the **bottom of your rib cage**.

Navel

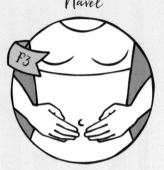

Close your eyes and cup your hands. With your palms facing you and your fingertips pointing toward each other, place your hands on your **middle abdomen**. Gently press your palms just below the **navel**.

Waist

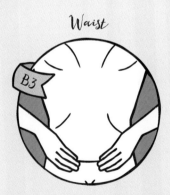

Close your eyes and cup your hands. With your palms facing you and your fingertips pointing toward each other, place your hands behind you, on the **lower part of your back**. Gently press the base of your palms on your **waist**.

PELVIS

Self Help

Groin

Coccyx

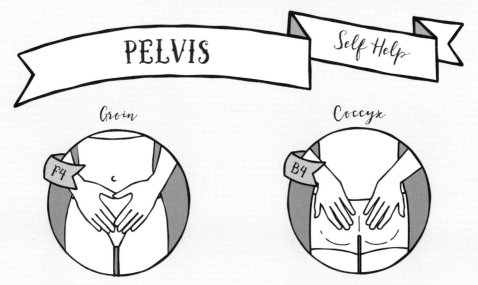

Close your eyes and cup your hands. With your palms facing you and your fingertips facing downward and inward, place your hands on your **lower abdomen**. Gently press the base of your palms on your **hips**.

Close your eyes and cup your hands. With your palms facing you and your fingertips pointing downward and inward, place your hands behind you, on the **top and center of your buttocks**. Gently press your little fingers on your **sacrum**.

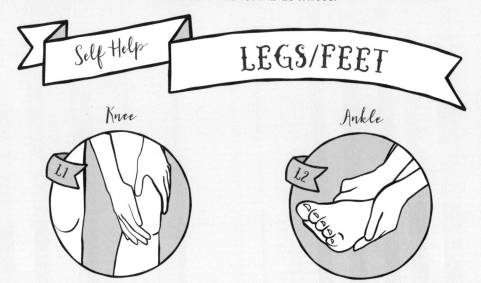

Self Help

LEGS/FEET

Knee

Close your eyes and cup your hands. Place the palm of your hand just above your **knee**. Place the palm of your other hand just below your **knee**.

Ankle

Close your eyes and cross your legs. Place your **ankle** on your **knee**. Cup your hands, placing them around your **ankle**.

Sole

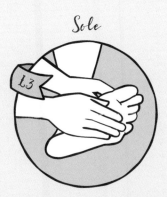

Close your eyes and cross your legs. Place your **ankle** on your **knee**. Cup your hands and place the palm of one hand on **top of the instep**. Place the other palm **under the arch on the sole of your foot**, with your thumbs touching, **just below your big toe**.

HEAD AND NECK

Family Help

Eyes

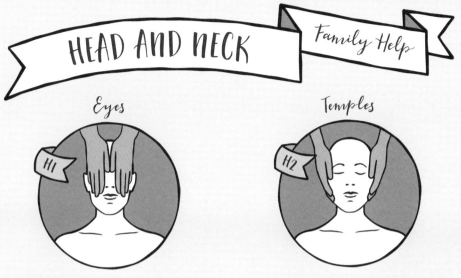

Cup your hands, with the sides of your thumbs touching and your fingers facing away from you. Gently place the base of your palms on the **top of the forehead**. Hover over the **eyes** and **cheeks**.

Temples

Cup your hands, with your fingers facing away from you. Gently place the base of your palms on the **sides of the forehead**. Hover over the **temples, ears,** and **side of the face**.

Skull

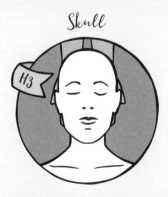

Cup your hands, with the sides of your little fingers touching. Have the receiver lift his or her **head** momentarily and cup the **head** in your hands. Gently hold the **back of the skull** in the palms of your hands.

Throat

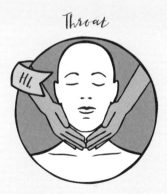

Cup your hands, with your index and middle fingers touching. Place the sides of your thumbs along the edge of the **jaw**. Hover over the **throat**.

Family Help

CHEST

Heart

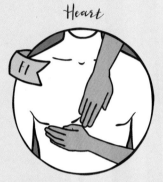

Shoulders

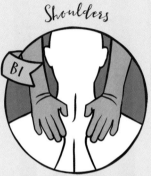

Ribs

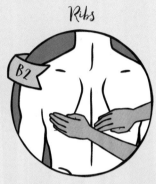

Cup your hands and place them perpendicular to each other. Face your palms downward, with the fingertips of one hand facing the feet and the fingertips of the other facing away from you. With the fingertips of the upper hand touching the side of the thumb of the other, hover over the **sternum** and the **bottom of the rib cage**.

Cup your hands and face your palms downward. Point your fingertips downward toward the feet and inward toward the **spine**. Gently place your hands on the **shoulders**.

Cup your hands and place them in tandem, with your fingertips facing away from you. With the fingertips of the hand closest to you, barely touch the palm of the hand farthest from you. Gently place your hands on the **shoulder blades** on the upper back.

UPPER ABDOMEN

Family Help

Solar Plexus

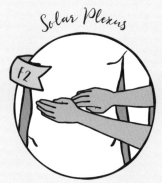

Navel

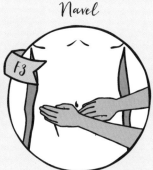

Waist

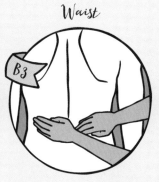

Cup your hands and place them in tandem, with your fingertips facing away from you. With the fingertips of the hand closest to you, barely touch the palm of the hand farthest from you. Hover over the **lower ribs** and the **upper abdomen**.

Cup your hands and place them in tandem, with your fingertips facing away from you. With the fingertips of the hand closest to you, barely touch the palm of the hand farthest from you. Hover over the **navel** and the **middle of the abdomen**.

Cup your hands and place them in tandem, with your fingertips facing away from you. With the fingertips of the hand closest to you, barely touch the palm of the hand farthest from you. Gently place your hands over the **mid-back**, at the lowest part of the rib cage.

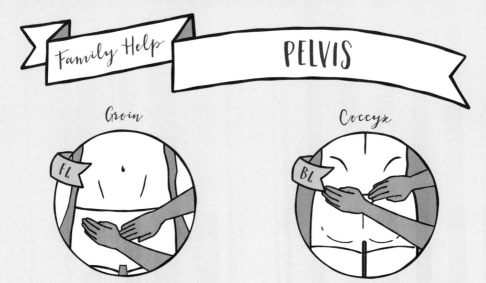

Family Help

PELVIS

Groin

Coccyx

Cup your hands and place them in tandem, with your fingertips facing away from you. With the fingertips of the hand closest to you, barely touch the palm of the hand farthest from you and form a V-shape. Hover over the **groin**, leaving at least 2 inches (6 centimeters) between you and the receiver.

Cup your hands and place them in tandem, with your fingertips facing away from you. With the fingertips of the hand closest to you, barely touch the palm of the hand farthest from you. Gently place your hands over the **lowest part of the spine**, just below the waist.

LEGS/FEET

Family Help

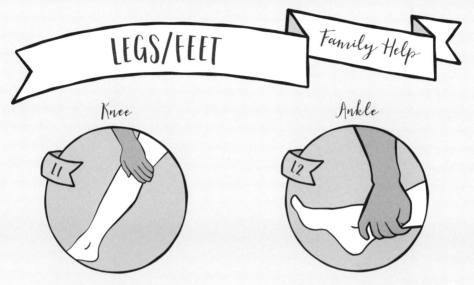

Knee

Cup your hands. Place the palm of one hand on **top of the kneecap**. Place the palm of the other hand **under the knee**.

Ankle

Cup your hands. Place the palm of one hand on **top of the ankle**. Place the palm of the other hand on the **other side of the ankle**.

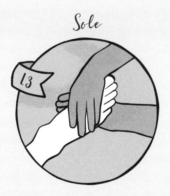

Sole

Cup your hands. Place the palm of one hand on **top of the instep of the foot**. Place the palm of the other hand **under the arch on the sole of the foot**.

AILMENTS BY BODY SYSTEM

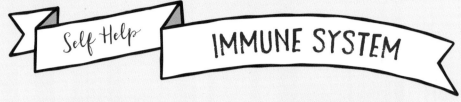

IMMUNE SYSTEM

Self Help

Heart

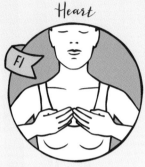

F1

Solar Plexus

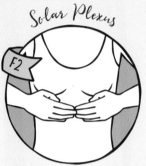

F2

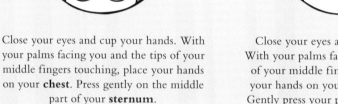

Close your eyes and cup your hands. With your palms facing you and the tips of your middle fingers touching, place your hands on your **chest**. Press gently on the middle part of your **sternum**.

Close your eyes and cup your hands. With your palms facing you and the tips of your middle fingers touching, place your hands on your **upper abdomen**. Gently press your palms on the **bottom of your rib cage**.

CIRCULATORY SYSTEM *Self Help*

Heart

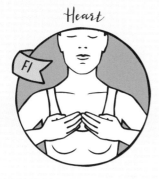

Shoulders

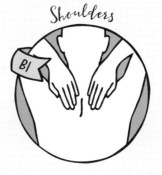

Close your eyes and cup your hands. With your palms facing you and the tips of your middle fingers touching, place your hands on your **chest**. Press gently on the middle part of your **sternum**.

Close your eyes and cup your hands. Place your hands behind you on the middle part of your **shoulders**, with your fingertips facing downward and inward, toward your **spine**. Gently press your fingers on your **shoulders**.

Self Help — GASTROINTESTINAL SYSTEM

Solar Plexus

Navel

Groin

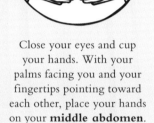

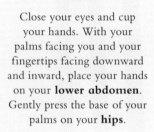

Close your eyes and cup your hands. With your palms facing you and the tips of your middle fingers touching, place your hands on your **upper abdomen**. Gently press your palms on the bottom of your **rib cage**.

Close your eyes and cup your hands. With your palms facing you and your fingertips pointing toward each other, place your hands on your **middle abdomen**. Gently press just below the **navel**.

Close your eyes and cup your hands. With your palms facing you and your fingertips facing downward and inward, place your hands on your **lower abdomen**. Gently press the base of your palms on your **hips**.

Waist

Coccyx

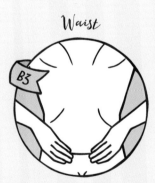

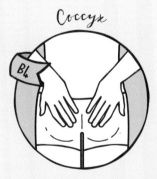

Close your eyes and cup your hands. With your palms facing you and your fingertips pointing toward each other, place your hands behind you, on the **lower part of your back.** Gently press the base of your palms on your **waist**.

Close your eyes and cup your hands. With your palms facing you and your fingertips pointing downward and inward, place your hands behind you, on the **top and center of your buttocks**. Gently press your little fingers on your **sacrum**.

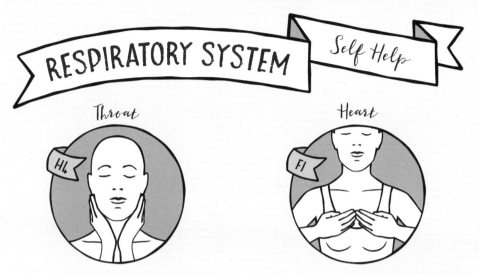

RESPIRATORY SYSTEM

Self Help

Throat

Close your eyes and cup your hands. Place your hands at the **front of your throat**, with the base of your palms touching. Hover beneath your **jaw**.

Heart

Close your eyes and cup your hands. With your palms facing you and the tips of your middle fingers touching, place your hands on your **chest**. Press gently on the middle part of your **sternum**.

Shoulders

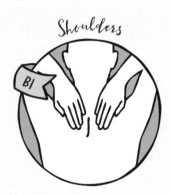

Close your eyes and cup your hands. Place your hands behind you on the middle part of your **shoulders**, with your fingertips facing downward and inward, toward your **spine**. Gently press your fingers on your **shoulders**.

Self Help ENDOCRINE SYSTEM

Temples

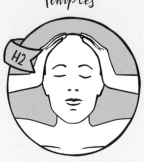

Close your eyes and cup
your hands. Hover your
hands over your **temples/
ears.** With your fingertips,
lightly touch the **side of
your forehead**.

Throat

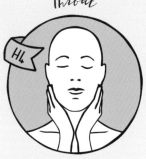

Close your eyes and cup
your hands. Place your
hands at the **front of your
throat**, with the base of
your palms touching. Hover
beneath your **jaw**.

Heart

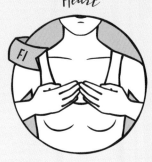

Close your eyes and cup
your hands. With your palms
facing you and the tips
of your middle fingers
touching, place your hands
on your **chest**. Press gently
on the middle part of
your **sternum**.

Solar Plexus

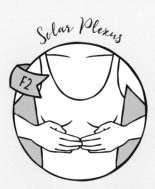

Close your eyes and cup your hands. With
your palms facing you and the tips of your
middle fingers touching, place your hands
on your **upper abdomen**. Gently press
your palms on the bottom of your
rib cage.

Groin

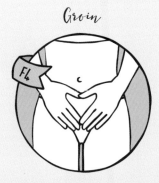

Close your eyes and cup your hands. With
your palms facing you and your fingertips
facing downward and inward, place your
hands on your **lower abdomen**. Gently
press the base of your palms on your **hips**.

IMMUNE SYSTEM

Family Help

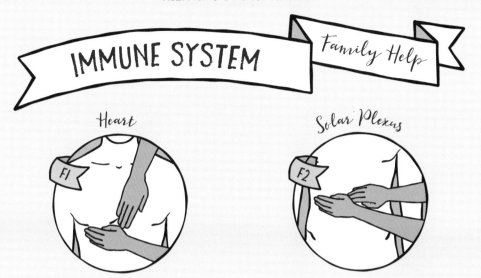

Heart

Solar Plexus

Cup your hands and place them perpendicular to each other. Face your palms downward, with the fingertips of one hand facing the feet and the fingertips of the other facing away from you. With the fingertips of the upper hand touching the side of the thumb of the other hand, hover over the **sternum** and the **bottom of the rib cage**.

Cup your hands and place them in tandem, with your fingertips facing away from you. With the fingertips of the hand closest to you, barely touch the palm of the hand farthest from you. Hover over the **lower ribs** and the **upper abdomen**.

CIRCULATORY SYSTEM

Heart

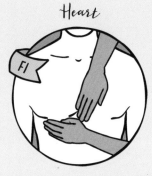

Ribs

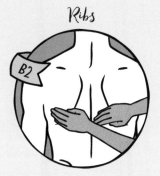

Cup your hands and place them perpendicular to each other. Face your palms downward, with the fingertips of one hand facing the feet and the fingertips of the other facing away from you. With the base of the upper hand touching the side of the thumb of the other hand, hover over the **sternum** and the **bottom of the rib cage**.

Cup your hands and place them in tandem, with your fingertips facing away from you. With the fingertips of the hand closest to you, barely touch the palm of the hand farthest from you. Gently place your hands on the **shoulder blades** on the upper back.

GASTROINTESTINAL SYSTEM
Family Help

Solar Plexus

F2

Cup your hands and place them in tandem, with your fingertips facing away from you. With the fingertips of the hand closest to you, barely touch the palm of the hand farthest from you. Hover over the **lower ribs** and the **upper abdomen**.

Navel

F3

Cup your hands and place them in tandem, with your fingertips facing away from you. With the fingertips of the hand closest to you, barely touch the palm of the hand farthest from you. Hover over the **navel** and the **middle of the abdomen**.

Groin

F4

Cup your hands and place them in tandem, with your fingertips facing away from you. With the fingertips of the hand closest to you, barely touch the palm of the hand farthest from you and form a V-shape. Hover over the **groin**.

Waist

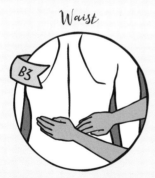

B3

Cup your hands and place them in tandem, with your fingertips facing away from you. With the fingertips of the hand closest to you, barely touch the palm of the hand farthest from you. Gently place your hands over the **mid-back**, at the lowest part of the rib cage.

Coccyx

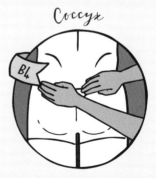

B4

Cup your hands and place them in tandem, with your fingertips facing away from you. With the fingertips of the hand closest to you, barely touch the palm of the hand farthest from you. Gently place your hands over the **lowest part of the spine**, just below the waist.

Family Help

RESPIRATORY SYSTEM

Throat

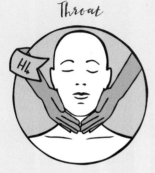

Cup your hands, with your index and middle fingers touching. Place the side of your thumbs along the edge of the **jaw**. Hover over the **throat**.

Heart

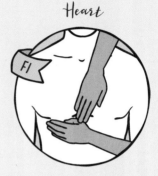

Cup your hands and place them perpendicular to each other. Face your palms downward, with the fingertips of one hand facing the feet and the fingertips of the other facing away from you. With the fingertips of the upper hand touching the thumb of the other, hover over the **sternum** and **bottom of the rib cage**.

Shoulders

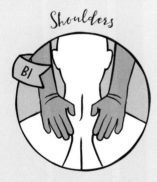

Cup your hands and face your palms downward. Point your fingertips downward toward the feet and inward toward the **spine**. Gently place your hands on the **shoulders**.

Ribs

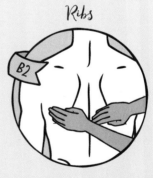

Cup your hands and place them in tandem, with your fingertips facing away from you. With the fingertips of the hand closest to you, barely touch the palm of the hand farthest from you. Gently place your hands on the **shoulder blades** on the upper back.

ENDOCRINE SYSTEM

Family Help

Temples

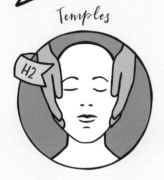

Cup your hands, with your fingers facing away from you. Gently place the base of your palms on the **sides of the forehead**. Hover over the **temples, ears**, and the **side of the face**.

Throat

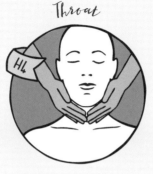

Cup your hands, with your index and middle fingers touching. Place the sides of your thumbs along the edge of the **jaw**. Hover over the **throat**.

Heart

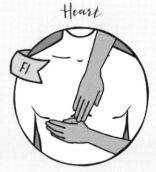

Cup your hands and place them perpendicular to each other. With the fingertips of the upper hand touching the thumb of the other, hover over the **sternum** and the **bottom of the rib cage**.

Solar Plexus

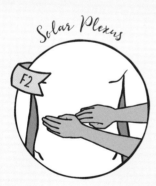

Cup your hands and place them in tandem, with your fingertips facing away from you. With the fingertips of the hand closest to you, barely touch the palm of the hand farthest from you. Hover over the **lower ribs** and the **upper abdomen**.

Groin

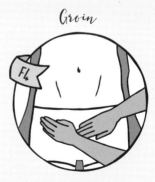

Cup your hands and place them in tandem, with your fingertips facing away from you. With the fingertips of the hand closest to you, barely touch the palm of the hand farthest from you and form a V-shape. Hover over the **groin**.

AILMENTS BY CHAKRA

BALANCING THE ROOT CHAKRA

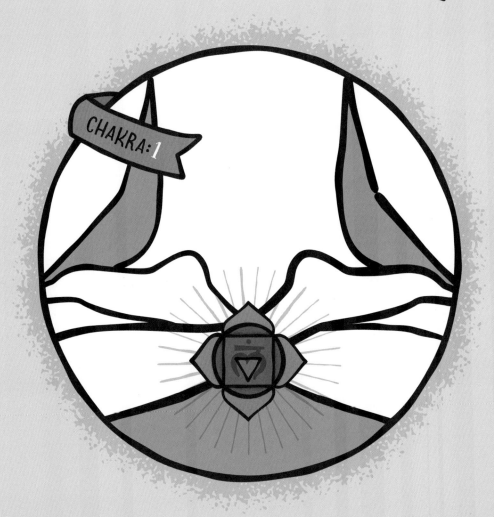

CHAKRA: 1

BALANCING THE ROOT CHAKRA

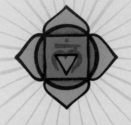

Begin long and deep breathing, and visualize the Reiki
Universal Life Energy flowing from the palms of your hands toward
the **base of your abdomen**. Using your mind's eye, "see" the
color RED spinning between your **genitals** and your **anus**. This
is your connection to the physical world. Trust and security rest
here. Allow this energy to ground and center you, leaving you
feeling at peace and whole.

Chakra: 1: Root

Color: Red

Location: Between genitals
and anus

Purpose: Links the individual
with the physical world

Element: Earth

Sense: Smell

Effect: Calms, dissolves tension

Body Parts: Bones, teeth,
nails, legs, arms, intestine, anus,
prostate, blood, cell structure,
adrenal gland

Tone: C

Zodiac & Planets: Aries,
Taurus, Scorpio,
Capricorn, Mars, Saturn

Groin

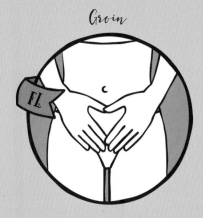

Coccyx

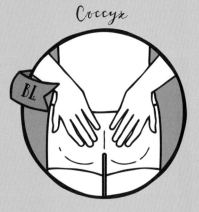

Close your eyes and cup your hands. With your palms facing you and your fingertips facing downward and inward, place your hands on your **lower abdomen**. Gently press the base of your palms on your **hips**.

Close your eyes and cup your hands. With your palms facing you and your fingertips pointing downward and inward, place your hands behind you, on the **top and center of your buttocks**. Gently press your little fingers on your **sacrum**.

BALANCING THE ROOT CHAKRA

Family Help

Groin

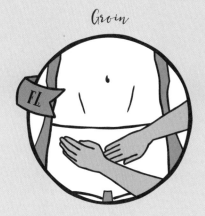

Coccyx

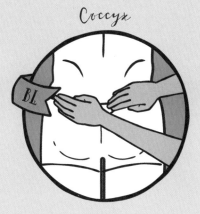

Cup your hands and place them in tandem, with your fingertips facing away from you. With the fingertips of the hand closest to you, barely touch the palm of the hand farthest from you and form a V-shape. Hover over the **groin**, leaving at least 2 inches (6 centimeters) between you and the receiver.

Cup your hands and place them in tandem, with your fingertips facing away from you. With the fingertips of the hand closest to you, barely touch the palm of the hand farthest from you. Gently place your hands over the **lowest part of the spine**, just below the waist.

BALANCING THE SACRAL CHAKRA

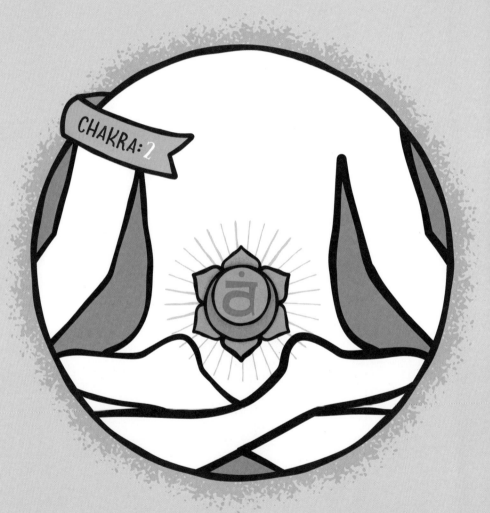

CHAKRA: 2

BALANCING THE SACRAL CHAKRA

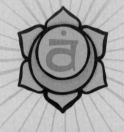

Begin long and deep breathing, and visualize the Reiki Universal Life Energy flowing from the palms of your hands toward the **center of your body**. Using your mind's eye, "see" the color ORANGE spinning just **below your navel**. This is the source of your creativity and inspiration. Your sexual desire and passion are born here. Allow your energy to flow freely, with joy and respect for your gift of creation.

Chakra: 2: Sacral

Color: Orange

Location: Slightly above genital area below navel

Purpose: Center for sexual energy, creativity, and pure emotions

Element: Water

Sense: Taste

Effect: Stimulates desire, rejuvenates

Body Parts: Reproductive organs, kidney, bladder, pelvic area, sperm, all liquids and fluids of the body

Tone: D

Zodiac & Planets: Cancer, Libra, Scorpio; Mercury, Venus, Moon, Mars

Groin

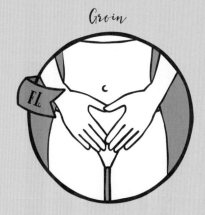

Coccyx

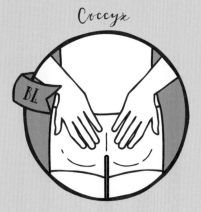

Close your eyes and cup your hands. With your palms facing you and your fingertips facing downward and inward, place your hands on your **lower abdomen**. Gently press the base of your palms on your **hips**.

Close your eyes and cup your hands. With your palms facing you and your fingertips pointing downward and inward, place your hands behind you, on the **top and center of your buttocks**. Gently press your little fingers on your **sacrum**.

BALANCING THE SACRAL CHAKRA

Family Help

Groin

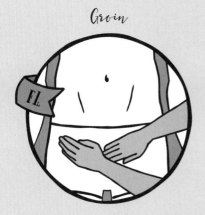

Coccyx

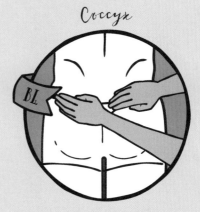

Cup your hands and place them in tandem, with your fingertips facing away from you. With the fingertips of the hand closest to you, barely touch the palm of the hand farthest from you and form a V-shape. Hover over the **groin**, leaving at least 2 inches (6 centimeters) between you and the receiver.

Cup your hands and place them in tandem, with your fingertips facing away from you. With the fingertips of the hand closest to you, barely touch the palm of the hand farthest from you. Gently place your hands over the **lowest part of the spine**, just below the waist.

BALANCING THE SOLAR-PLEXUS CHAKRA

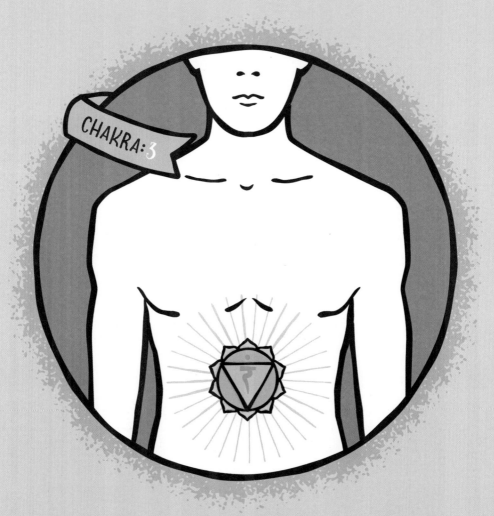

CHAKRA: 3

BALANCING THE SOLAR-PLEXUS CHAKRA

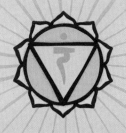

Begin long and deep breathing, and visualize the Reiki Universal Life Energy flowing from the palms of your hands toward the **center of your body**. Using your mind's eye, "see" the color YELLOW spinning in your **solar plexus**. This is core of your power, the source of your wisdom, and your "gut feeling", where the upper and lower chakras are balanced and integrated. Allow this balancing and integrating to occur.

Chakra: 3: Solar plexus

Color: Yellow

Location: Slightly up from the navel

Purpose: This is where the personality is formed. Feeling and being are integrated here

Element: Fire

Sense: Sight

Effect: Eases aggression, pacifies

Body Parts: Abdomen, lower back, stomach, spleen, liver, digestive system, gallbladder, autonomic nervous system, pancreas

Tone: E

Zodiac & Planets: Leo, Virgo, Sagittarius; Sun, Mercury, Mars, Jupiter

Navel

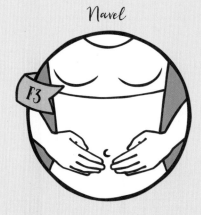

Waist

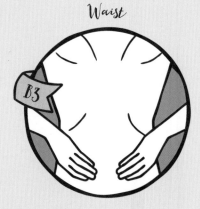

Close your eyes and cup your hands. With your palms facing you and your fingertips pointing toward each other, place your hands on your **middle abdomen**. Gently press just below the **navel**.

Close your eyes and cup your hands. With your palms facing you and your fingertips pointing toward each other, place your hands behind you, on the **lower part of your back**. Gently press the base of your palms on your **waist**.

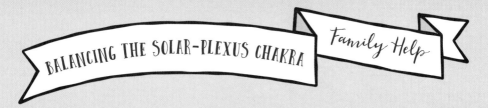

BALANCING THE SOLAR-PLEXUS CHAKRA   *Family Help*

Navel

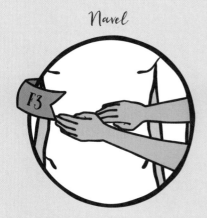

Waist

Cup your hands and place them in tandem, with your fingertips facing away from you. With the fingertips of the hand closest to you, barely touch the palm of the hand farthest from you. Hover over the **lower ribs** and the **upper abdomen**.

Cup your hands and place them in tandem, with your fingertips facing away from you. With the fingertips of the hand closest to you, barely touch the palm of the hand farthest from you. Gently place your hands over the **mid-back**, at the lowest part of the rib cage.

BALANCING THE HEART CHAKRA

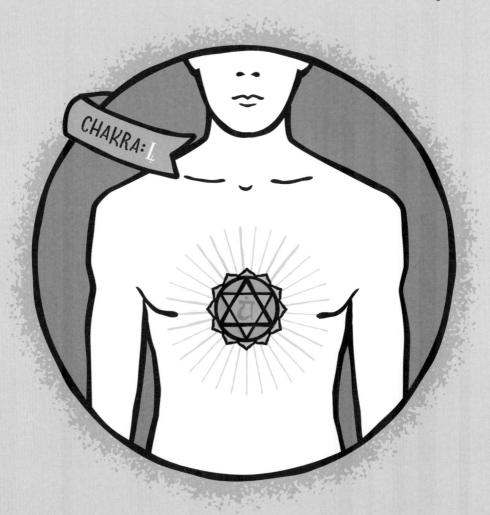

CHAKRA: L

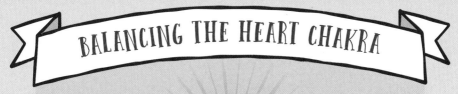

BALANCING THE HEART CHAKRA

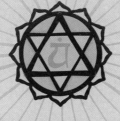

Begin long and deep breathing, and visualize the Reiki Universal Life Energy flowing from the palms of your hands toward the **center of your body**. Using your mind's eye, "see" the color GREEN spinning in your **heart**. This is the source of your ability to love and to heal. Allow this energy to generate gratitude, with great compassion for yourself and great empathy for others.

Chakra: 4: Heart

Color: Green

Location: Center of chest

Purpose: The ability to love without fear and self-consciousness

Element: Air

Sense: Touch

Effect: Brings peace and understanding

Body Parts: Heart, upper back, rib cage, chest, skin, circulatory system, lower lungs, abdominal cavity, thymus gland

Tone: F

Zodiac & Planets: Leo, Libra, Sun, Venus, Saturn

Heart

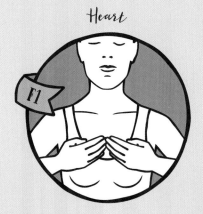

Shoulders

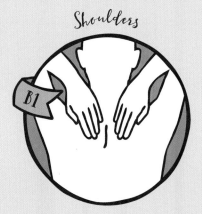

Close your eyes and cup your hands. With your palms facing you and the tips of your middle fingers touching, place your hands on your **chest**. Press gently on the middle part of your **sternum**.

Close your eyes and cup your hands. Place your hands behind you on the middle part of your **shoulders**, with your fingertips facing downward and inward, toward your **spine**. Gently press your fingers on your **shoulders**.

BALANCING THE HEART CHAKRA

Family Help

Heart

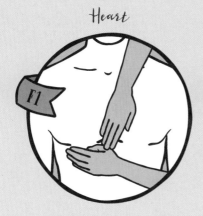

Shoulders

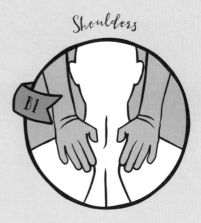

Cup your hands and place them perpendicular to each other. Face your palms downward, with the fingertips of one hand facing the feet and the fingertips of the other facing away from you. With the fingertips of the upper hand touching the side of the thumb of the other hand, hover over the **sternum** and the **bottom of the rib cage**.

Cup your hands and face your palms downward. Point your fingertips downward toward the **feet** and inward toward the **spine**. Gently place your hands on the **shoulders**.

BALANCING THE THROAT CHAKRA

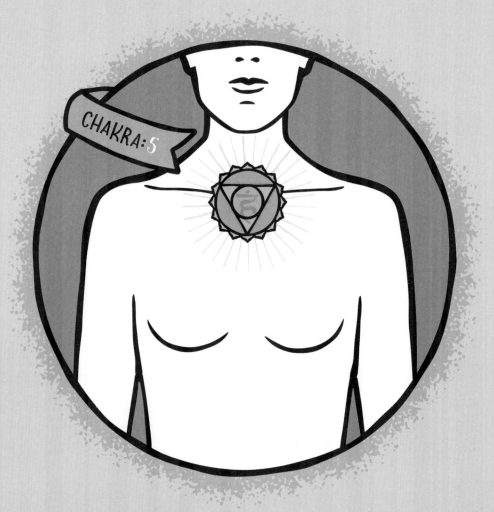

CHAKRA: 5

BALANCING THE THROAT CHAKRA

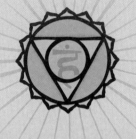

Begin long and deep breathing, and visualize the Reiki
Universal Life Energy flowing from the palms of your hands toward
your **throat**. Using your mind's eye, "see" the color LIGHT BLUE
spinning in your **neck**. This is the source of your voice and self
expression. Allow this energy to give you confidence to
communicate who you are to the world, and to share
your inspiration with others.

Chakra: 5: Throat

Color: Light blue

Location: Between inner
collarbone

Purpose: Deals with all
related to sound, both physical
and metaphysical

Element: Ether

Sense: Sound

Effect: Brings harmony to
speech and voice

Body Parts: Lungs, vocal
chords, bronchi, throat, jaw, neck,
thyroid, voice, nape of neck,
thyroid gland

Tone: G

Zodiac & Planets: Taurus,
Gemini, Aquarius; Venus, Mars,
Uranus

Self Help

BALANCING THE THROAT CHAKRA

Throat

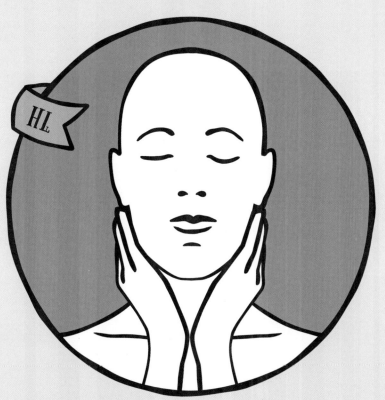

Close your eyes and cup your hands. Place your hands at the **front of your throat**, with the base of your palms touching. Hover beneath your **jaw**.

BALANCING THE THROAT CHAKRA

Family Help

Throat

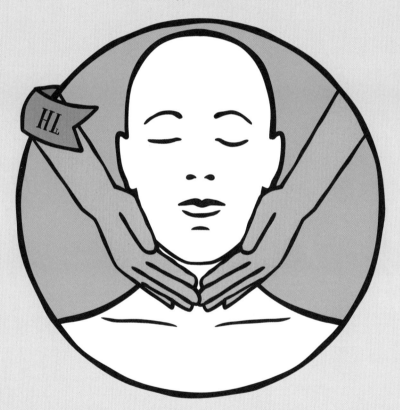

Cup your hands, with your index and middle fingers touching. Place the
sides of your thumbs along the edge of the **jaw**. Hover over the **throat**.

BALANCING THE THIRD-EYE CHAKRA

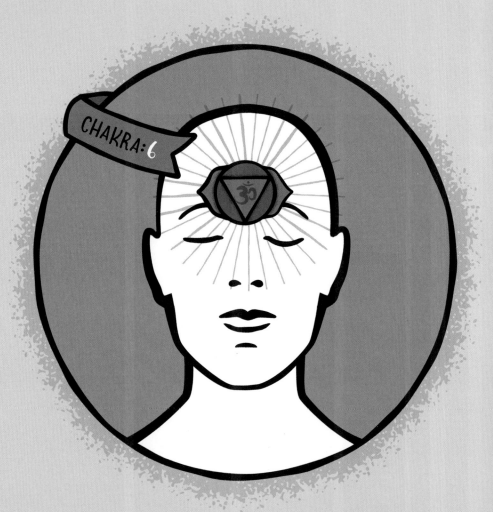

CHAKRA: 6

BALANCING THE THIRD-EYE CHAKRA

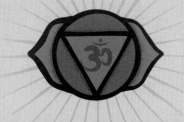

Begin long and deep breathing, and visualize the Reiki Universal Life Energy flowing from the palms of your hands toward the **center of your forehead**, between and just above your eyebrows. Using your mind's eye, "see" the color INDIGO spinning in your **forehead**. This is the source of your inner vision—your intuition and awareness of self. Allow this energy to inform and bring harmony to your understanding of the world.

Chakra: 6: Third Eye

Color: Indigo

Location: Between the eyes

Purpose: This chakra enables the recognition of being

Element: All elements

Sense: All plus sixth sense

Effect: Understanding, harmony

Body Parts: Face, nose, eyes, sinus, cerebellum, pituitary gland

Tone: A

Zodiac & Planets: Sagittarius, Aquarius, Pisces, Mercury, Venus, Uranus

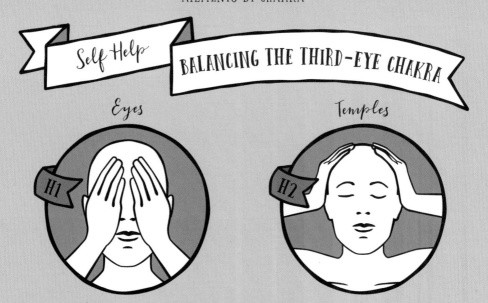

Self Help

BALANCING THE THIRD-EYE CHAKRA

Eyes

H1

Close your eyes and cup your hands. Hover your hands over your **eyes**. With your fingertips, lightly touch the **top of your forehead**.

Temples

H2

Close your eyes and cup your hands. Hover your hands over your **temples/ears**. With your fingertips, lightly touch the **side of your forehead**.

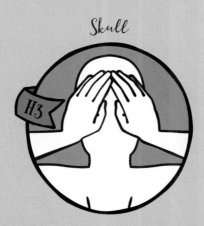

Skull

H3

Close your eyes and place your hands on the **back of your skull**. Touch your index and middle fingers together. Hover your hands over the **back and lower part of your skull**.

BALANCING THE THIRD-EYE CHAKRA *Family Help*

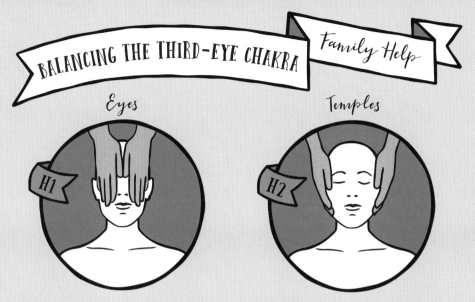

Eyes

H1

Cup your hands, with the sides of your thumbs touching and your fingers facing away from you. Gently place the base of your palms on the **top of the forehead**. Hover over the **eyes** and **cheeks**.

Temples

H2

Cup your hands, with your fingers facing away from you. Gently place the base of your palms on the **sides of the forehead**. Hover over the **ears** and the **side of the face**.

Skull

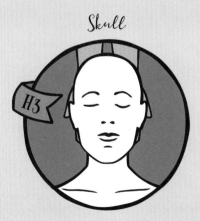

H3

Cup your hands, with the sides of your little fingers touching. Have the receiver lift his or her **head** momentarily and cup the head in your hands. Gently hold the **back of the skull** in the palms of your hands.

BALANCING THE CROWN CHAKRA

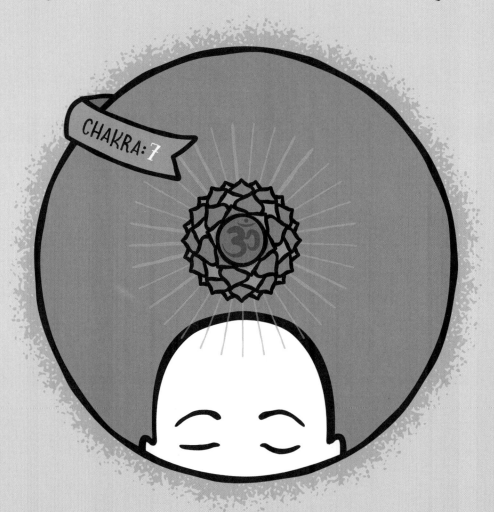

CHAKRA: 7

BALANCING THE CROWN CHAKRA

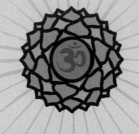

Begin long and deep breathing, and visualize the Reiki Universal Life Energy flowing from the palms of your hands, through your **fingers**, toward the **top of your head**. Using your mind's eye, "see" the color VIOLET or WHITE spinning at the **crown of your head**. This is the point of connection to the divine through your higher self. Allow this energy to bring you deep peace and joy, and enter you into a state of infinite possibilities.

Chakra: 7: Crown

Color: Violet, white

Location: Top and center of head

Purpose: Here the human being connects with the universe

Element: All elements

Sense: Beyond senses

Effect: Cosmic aspect—no self limitations

Body Parts: Brain, cerebellum, skull, pineal gland

Tone: Hum

Zodiac & Planets: Capricorn, Pisces, Saturn, Neptune

Self Help

BALANCING THE CROWN CHAKRA

Eyes

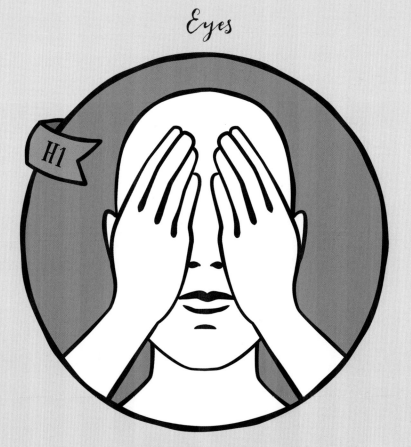

Close your eyes and cup your hands. Hover your hands over your **eyes**. With your fingertips, lightly touch the **top of your forehead**.

BALANCING THE CROWN CHAKRA

Family Help

Eyes

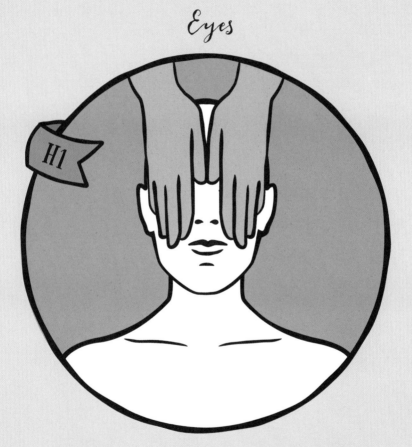

Cup your hands, with the sides of your thumbs touching and your
fingers facing away from you. Gently place the base of your palms on
the **top of the forehead**. Hover over the **eyes** and **cheeks**.

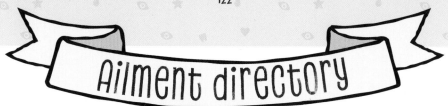

Ailment directory

Reiki can be beneficial for a wide variety of health issues, easing pain and discomfort, as well as helping to reduce or eliminate other symptoms. Each ailment in this alphabetically organized list is followed by the hand positions you can work for relief.

AILMENT	DESCRIPTION	SELF-HELP HAND POSITIONS	FAMILY-HELP HAND POSITIONS
Adrenal fatigue	Prolonged stress can cause the adrenal glands to fatigue and cause a variety of symptoms, from tiredness to weight gain.	F2, B2	F2, B3
Allergies	The liver cleanses the blood of toxins and chemical buildup, which may contribute to allergies.	H1, H3, F2, B2	H1, H3, F2, B3
Anxiety	Relaxing the diaphragm muscle can help us to breathe more easily.	H3, F3, B3	H3, F2, B3
Arthritis	For pain and stiffness associated with arthritis use hand positions corresponding to the affected body part.	H1, H3, F2, B2 + Specific location (LOC)	H1, H3, F2, B3 + Specific LOC
Asthma	It is important to help the lungs and bronchial tubes to relax, which may help to ease labored breathing.	F1, F2, B1, B2	H4, F1, F2, B1, B2, B3
Bronchitis	Bronchitis symptoms include cough, chest discomfort, and shortness of breath.	F1, F2, B1, B2	H4, F1, F2, B1, B2, B3
Bursitis (knee, elbow, or shoulder)	Bursitis is an inflammation of the fluid-filled sac in the knee, elbow, or shoulder joints.	H1, H3, F2, B2 + Specific LOC	H1, H3, F2, B3 + Specific LOC
Crohn's disease	Crohn's disease is an inflammatory bowel disease that can affect different areas of the digestive tract.	F3, B3	F2, F3
Cold/Flu	Helping the immune system to work more efficiently is key to getting over a cold or flu faster.	Standard overall or Specific LOC	Standard overall or Specific LOC
Constipation	Constipation often means that the digestive tract is not working efficiently.	F2, F3, F4, B2, B3	F2, F3, F4, B3
Depression	A relaxing and soothing standard overall session can help a person feel better.	H1-H3 or standard overall	H1-H4 or standard overall

AILMENT	DESCRIPTION	SELF-HELP HAND POSITIONS	FAMILY-HELP HAND POSITIONS
Dermatitis (atopic/eczema)	For symptoms of itching, redness, and dry skin, use hand positions corresponding to the affected body part.	Standard overall or Specific LOC	Standard overall or Specific LOC
Diabetes	In some forms of diabetes, the pancreas is not producing enough insulin, which is responsible for decreasing blood sugar (glucose).	F2, B2	F2, B3
Diarrhea	When experiencing the discomforts of diarrhea, use hand positions corresponding to the upper-, mid-, and lower-abdomen.	F3, F4, B3, B4	F2, F3, F4, B3, B4
Diverticulitis	Diverticulitis is an inflammatory disease, which can affect the sigmoid colon with symptoms such as pain, nausea, and disturbance of bowel function.	F2, F4, B4	F2, F4, B4
Dizziness and other inner ear problems	Dizziness is often caused by imbalance of the inner ear.	H2, H3	H2, H3
Ear infection	Ear infections can be very painful.	H2, H4, F1	H2, H4, F1
Elbow pain and tennis elbow (epicondylitis)	Epicondylitis can be caused by irritation of the tissue connecting forearm muscle to the elbow.	Standard overall or Specific LOC	Standard overall or Specific LOC
Eye fatigue	One of the most common causes of eye fatigue is staring too long at digital devices.	H1, H2	H1, H2
Gastritis	Gastritis is an inflammation of the stomach lining.	F2, B2	F2, B3
Gallstones	The gallbladder plays an important role in regulating cholesterol.	F2, B2	F2, B3
Headache	Headache pain can have a variety of causes and can be felt in different areas of your head.	H1–H3, B1	H1–H4, B1
Heartburn (acid reflux)	When suffering from acid reflux, you might feel discomfort in the chest when acid travels up from the stomach through the esophagus.	F2, B2	F2, B3
Hiatal hernia	A hiatal hernia is caused by part of the stomach bulging through the diaphragm muscle.	F2, B2	F2, B3
Hiccups	Hiccups are sudden spasms of the diaphragm muscle.	F2, B2	F2, B3
High blood pressure (hypertension)	It is important to relax the entire body of a person who experiences high blood pressure.	F1, F2, B1, B2	F1, F2, B2, B3

AILMENT	DESCRIPTION	SELF-HELP HAND POSITIONS	FAMILY-HELP HAND POSITIONS
Hip pain	For any hip pain, use hand positions corresponding to the affected areas.	F4, L1	F4, L1
Inguinal hernia	An inguinal hernia can cause severe pain from the weakened abdominal wall.	F3, F4, B3	F3, F4, B4
Irritable bowel syndrome (IBS)	IBS is an intestinal disorder with symptoms such as nausea, bloating, abdominal cramping, diarrhea, and constipation.	F3, F4, B3, B4	F2, F3, F4, B3, B4
Jaw tension and temporomandibular joint (TMJ) disorder	TMJ disorder can cause pain in the jaw joint and muscles.	H3, H4	H2, H3
Kidney stones	Kidney stones are small, hard deposits of mineral and acid salts inside your kidneys.	F2, B2	F2, B3
Knee pain	For knee pain, use hand positions around the affected knee.	L1	L1
Leg pain and leg cramps	If you experience pain from too much vigorous exercise, leg cramps or other causes of leg pain, use hand positions corresponding to the affected areas.	L1-L3	L1-L3
Lower back pain and stiffness (lumbago)	For lower back pain and stiffness, it is helpful to relax the muscles attached to the lumbar spine in addition to relaxing the broader lumbar area.	F3, F4, B3, B4	F3, F4, B3, B4
Migraines	When suffering from migraines, use hand positions corresponding to the head.	H1-H3, B1	H1-H4, B1
Morning sickness	Many women suffer from nausea in the first trimester of pregnancy.	F2, B2	F2, B3
Nausea	Nausea of any kind can be helped by using the hand positions corresponding to the diaphragm, solar plexus, and stomach.	F2, B2	F2, B3
Neck pain and stiff neck	To ease neck tension, pain, and stiffness, it is helpful to use the hand positions corresponding to the affected area.	H3, H4, B1	H3, H4, B1
Premenstrual syndrome and menstrual cramps	Premenstrual syndrome or PMS usually starts about one week before menstruation.	H1, F4, B4	H1, F4, B4

AILMENT	DESCRIPTION	SELF-HELP HAND POSITIONS	FAMILY-HELP HAND POSITIONS
Prostate issues/ enlarged prostate	Many men, as they age, have an enlarged prostate, which may affect normal urination.	F4, B4	F4, B4
Psoriasis	Psoriasis, a chronic skin disorder, can cause itchy, red, raised, scaly patches to appear on the skin.	Standard overall or Specific LOC	Standard overall or Specific LOC
Sciatica	The sciatic nerve starts at the lower back and runs through the buttocks and down each leg.	F4, L1-L3, B4	F4, L1-L3, B4
Shoulder pain	Shoulder pain can be caused by a variety of issues, from injury and muscle tension to arthritis and more.	H3, H4, B1	H3, H4, B1, B2
Sinus congestion and sinusitis	From allergies to a cold, you can find relief by using the hand positions corresponding to the affected areas.	H1, H2	H1, H2
Sore throat and tonsillitis	A sore throat is often the first sign of a cold, whereas tonsillitis is an inflammation or infection of the tonsils at the back of the throat.	H4, F1, B1	H4, F1, B1
Stomach ache	Stomach pain can be caused by a variety of issues.	F2, B2	F2, B3
Thyroid dysfunction	The thyroid gland is located at the base of the neck and is essential for producing hormones that affect metabolism. Over-function or under-function of the thyroid gland is a common issue.	H1, H4	H1, H4
Tinnitus	Tinnitus is commonly referred to as ringing or buzzing in the ears and can be temporary or chronic.	H2-H4	H2-H4
Toothache	If the cause of the toothache is unknown, make sure to see a dentist.	H3, H4	H2, H3
Ulcer	Common symptoms of stomach ulcers are burning stomach pain, bloating, feeling of fullness, fatty food intolerance, and nausea.	F2, B2	F2, B3
Urinary tract infection (UTI)	The burning of a urinary tract infection can be very painful.	F4, B4	F4, B4

INDEX

ACKNOWLEDGMENTS

I stand on the shoulders of giants. I'd like to thank the following masters for their guidance and wisdom: Siri Gopal Singh, Krishna Kaur, Sangeet Kaur, Bill Flocco, Lisa Chan, Logan Griffin, and Gary Strauss. And special thanks to Stefanie Sabounchian for making this book possible.

I am forever grateful for the teachings that have inspired and enlightened my path. They include "Conversations with God," "A Course In Miracles," The Ageless Wisdom Teachings, Landmark Education, 3HO Foundation, American Academy of Reflexology, and Life Energy Institute.

I am also indebted to the following pillars of strength that have supported me on my journey—my parents, Porfirio and Orlinda Archuleta; my siblings, Viv, Mark, Polly, and Frances; and my best of besties, Tim, Chris, Michael, and Julie, who have always had my back.

I'd like to thank my amazing team at Quarto Publishing for making the writing of this book such a pleasure. "Ladies of London." et. al., you're awesome!

Last, and certainly not least, I'd like to thank my husband, Steven, for his undying support and belief in my greatness and for loving me unconditionally. You light up my life…

Peace to all,

Victor

FOR MY GUARDIAN ANGELS, MARGARET, MERCEDES, AND MONTY.